T0219454

The Open Door

Art and Foreign Policy at the RCSI

Edited by Kevin M. Cahill, M.D.

A Joint Publication of
The Royal College of Surgeons in Ireland and
The Center for International Humanitarian Cooperation
Dublin 2014

Published by The Royal College of Surgeons in Ireland (RCSI)
and The Center for International Humanitarian Cooperation (CIHC)

ISBN 978-0-8232-6399-8

Cover and book designed by Massimo Vignelli
Cover art by Louis Le Brocquy

The photos in this book were taken at the RCSI by the
College Photographer Bobby's Studio of Dublin at the time of
each Lecture, or are portraits provided by the speakers.
Photograph on back jacket flap by Mitch Epstein
Printed in Ireland by W & G Baird

Distributed in the United States by Fordham University Press
as part of the International Humanitarian Affairs Book Series

For All Healers and Peacemakers

Contents

Introduction

In 1852, the Reverend John Henry Newman delivered a series of lectures in Dublin calling for a comprehensive system of higher education to serve the Catholic population. In *The Idea of a University* he envisioned a medical school as the central priority, for, as he explained, all knowledge, in all the arts and sciences, should ultimately be for the benefit of mankind, and it was in the medical school where all aspects of the human being were studied and applied. Consequently, a medical school was opened on Cecilia Street in 1855 but, since it was not an officially recognized institution, The Royal College of Surgeons in Ireland (RCSI) conferred their degrees in the early years. Almost a century and a half later another remarkable series of lectures were delivered at RCSI.

This volume, *The Open Door: Art and Foreign Policy at the RCSI*, derives from those lectures delivered over a two decade period from 1986 to 2006. They reflect Newman's philosophy on the need to have a medical school that would be open to new ideas, constantly broadening the foundations – and the horizons – of medicine, and enabling us to share the ethos of our noble profession with others.

When I was appointed Professor and Chairman of the Department of Tropical Medicine in 1969, I faced many challenges in developing a new discipline in the RCSI, not least was in convincing academic colleagues on the significance of tropical medicine in a Dublin school, understandably focused on more traditional courses of concern in a European capital with no over-seas colonies. To secure an independent department, and adequate time in a crowded curriculum, were obvious early hurdles.

During my thirty-six year tenure as Professor and Chairman of the Department, I taught over four thousand medical students and hundreds of post-graduate candidates for specialty diplomas. The tropical medicine course at the RCSI became the most extensive undergraduate program in Europe and America, and a "stopping exam" assured the attention of sometimes reluctant students who could not proceed to their final year without passing our test. The Department attracted internationally renowned faculty. We created a tropical medicine museum, the first audio-visual section in the College, an international journal publication, a series of textbooks, and an overseas elective scheme for students. But by far the most inclusive and festive event in the Department calendar was our Annual Distinguished International Lecture, and this became an integral part of College life.

Using personal contacts (all Lecturers were patients and friends), and a modest endowment fund, I invited people who I believed would enrich the College by delivering a formal lecture, meeting with a small student seminar, and then enjoying the hospitality of a banquet in the elegant Board Room overlooking Stephen's Green. Although the lecture series began with professional colleagues discussing specific diseases, it soon reflected my interests in the role of health and humanitarian affairs in foreign policy and diplomacy, and then on the even broader impact of art and culture on our profession. The first edition of the book, *The Open Door: Health and Foreign Policy at the RCSI* was published in 1999; this second edition includes six later Lectures, and is presented in reverse chronological order with the most recent talk first and the earliest last.

Medicine has never been a pure science, primarily because it deals with populations that are not merely biological robots. Human beings are complex entities, influenced by traditions, cultures, emotions, and many other factors that affect the manifestations of disease and responses to therapy. All the non-medical Lecturers provided fresh thoughts for our consideration, but they also assured me that they too profited from the experience. Health professionals have the rarely recognized potential to influence public policy, and even provide great insights for an artist's search for meaning in life.

As I became more and more involved in humanitarian crises, particularly in conflict and post-conflict zones, I had to deal with the myriad of non-medical demands that flourish in the chaos of refugee camps. This new interest led to a series of invitations to Lecturers to come to the College and share their global perspective with our students, faculty and friends. Thus came to the RCSI, the Secretary of State of the United States of America, the Secretary-General of the United Nations, a Nobel Peace Laureate, the founder of an international non-governmental organization, the Foreign Ministers of the United Kingdom and Sweden, as well as a world famous neurologist/philosopher.

Most of the original contributors did not realize that the RCSI was then the most international medical school in the Western world, with students from 40 nations. The College, in the very heart of Dublin, had a mosque in the basement that served the spiritual needs of Islamic students. In our troubled world there was fertile soil in the College—a marvelous mixture of races, religions and cultures—that could be planted with imaginative initiatives, that were carefully nurtured till new programs evolved. The very title of the Department was changed to include the broader field of International Health. The Distinguished Lectures reflected an even broader vision for our noble and ancient profession. It was through our remarkable "open door" that Lecturers helped expand the traditional definition of medicine. I have kept the texts from the first edition unchanged for several reasons: even though some were written more than 20 years ago they are remarkably readable today as reflections on current diplomatic debates; also some of the authors have died or are ill, and it seemed inappropriate to edit some contributions and not others.

The Open Door: Art and Foreign Policy at the RCSI contains a new Foreword by the current President of the College, this revised Introduction, updated biographies and six additional chapters that emphasize the universal role of culture in humanity and healing. The first Lecture is by an internationally renowned French physician/activist/author/politician/diplomat. The following two chapters offer my own thoughts on assuming a new Professorship in the College and, in an earlier Distinguished Lecture, on the opportunities afforded when health and foreign policy are integrated.

The next two new contributions are by Irish artists—one a painter, and the other a poet—both dear friends who shared their own journeys of discovery with an audience that too rarely focused on "the whole thing," the "goodness" of sounds, the virtue of poetry, and of art, the "wholeness" and "whatness" of an image, and the quality of paint itself. Re-reading these texts brings back memorable talks by sublime artists, both sadly now dead. The next chapter in this book is a unique academic contribution by a former Taoiseach (Prime Minister) of Ireland who returned for the Lecture to his original profession as a demographer and statistician.

The next chapter is by a person of exceptional talent and passion;

she has been described as the "greatest actress of our generation." Her life has been an admirable mixture of theater and helping oppressed people all over the world. When performing in New York she would finish a show on Broadway, and travel out to the Queens House of Detention to see if she could help young women threatened by deportation. I was involved in many such efforts with Ms. Redgrave, linking medicine and art in very practical ways.

These new chapters complement the linkages between health, diplomacy and foreign affairs that were the primary focus of the first edition of this book. The new contributors suggest additional potential opportunities to realize the untapped resources that art and culture offer to our profession, and to all our inextricably shared lives. All the Distinguished Lecturers in this series graciously gave permission to publish the texts of their speeches in a planned collected volume; I express, once again, my gratitude to each of the contributors for sharing in this joint effort. The warmth and spontaneity of an oral presentation has been preserved by presenting, with minor grammatical corrections, the verbatim records of the Lectures. The two exceptions to this—as noted in their chapters—were by Ms. Redgrave where technical problems in the tape required a significant re-writing, and David Owen who updated some statistics and examples for the first edition of this book in 1999.

I wish to thank the Presidents of RCSI and the CEO's of the College with whom I have worked harmoniously and fruitfully for over 40 years. In particular, I acknowledge the cooperation and support throughout the decades of Harry O'Flanagan, Bill MacGowan, Kevin O'Malley, Michael Horgan, and Cathal Kelly. In preparing this new edition of *The Open Door: Art and Foreign Policy at the RCSI*, I had the great pleasure of once again working closely with Michael Horgan. His enthusiasm and practical assistance in assuring publication and offering editorial advice was deeply appreciated.

I acknowledge my thanks to the memory of Louis Le Brocquy for his India ink drawing of the College's main entrance as the "open door" that inspired the title of this volume.

Dermot Desmond, and his company, *Intuition Publishing*, generously provided transatlantic transportation and office support throughout this project.

My dear friend, Massimo Vignelli, designed both the cover and book layout for this edition; design production was provided by Mauro Sarri of Vignelli Associates.

Kevin M. Cahill, M.D.

Foreword

My predecessor, friend and mentor, Barry O'Donnell, in his Foreword for the first edition of *The Open Door,* summarised Kevin Cahill's career and interests as well as his contributions to humanitarianism and the development of the international health concept. Kevin served RCSI as Professor and Chairman of the Department of Tropical Medicine and International Health for thirty-six years until 2006, and was then appointed to a newly created Chair as Professor of International Humanitarian Affairs. The College has benefited hugely from the visits of the many world leaders who gave the Annual Distinguished International Lectures, and Kevin's continued energy and enthusiasm has resulted in this new and expanded edition now entitled, *The Open Door: Art & Foreign Policy*. I am honoured and delighted to be asked to write the Foreword to this book.

The open door is a very Irish concept. It implies a welcome to enter the home, or institution of the owner. In educational institutions an open door equates with an open mind, something that in my view is essential in our doctors and medical students of today. Even in the fifteen years that have elapsed since the first edition of this book, the level of extreme specialisation in medicine results in doctors working very much in their own contained silos. This collection of lectures and essays provides material for reflection on the wider issues that impact on health care delivery throughout the world as well as on the importance of art and culture in medicine.

My personal favourite is by our late lamented poet and Honorary Fellow of our own College, Seamus Heaney. His lecture on

"The Good of Poetry" was so interesting and challenging and so exemplifies his power of language that the entire lecture, or elements of it, should in my view be included in our undergraduate curriculum. Louis Le Brocquy's lecture on *"The Human Head: Notes on Painting and Awareness"* is also a fascinating insight into the mind of the artist and how differently to the rest of us they can perceive things. All 14 essays/lectures provide insights and detail to issues or stories that we may have glanced at in the foreign section of our newspapers. It is easy to visualise John Hume, Vanessa Redgrave, Garret FitzGerald and Aengus Finucane delivering their lectures on subjects about which they were so knowledgeable and so passionate.

Kevin Cahill deserves the gratitude and appreciation of RCSI, an institution he has served with distinction and dedication for so many years. His vision and understanding of the interactions between foreign policy, diplomacy, the arts and health and humanitarian affairs, is second to none.

Congratulations, Kevin, and thank you for allowing us to listen to many great leaders and visionaries under our own roof here in RCSI.

Patrick J. Broe, MCh FRCSI
President, Royal College of Surgeons in Ireland

Foreword to the First Edition

The sub-title *Health and Foreign Policy at the RCSI* is arresting; but then Professor Kevin Cahill, the Editor, is a remarkable man. He has impeccable Irish-American genes and upbringing (New York City) and has been in a sense playing a missionary role in the land of his fathers.

He is President and Director of the Center for International Humanitarian Cooperation as well as Director of the Tropical Disease Center at Lenox Hill Hospital in New York City. He holds teaching Chairs in Tropical Medicine at both New York University and the Royal College of Surgeons in Ireland. He sits on the Boards of a number of national and international charities. The United Nations Health Service has made him a Consultant in International Health. He is a polymath with a greatly developed sense of doing what he can for the public good. He may be classified as a patriot in both the United States and Ireland, and he is in the best sense a citizen of the world.

He correctly identified Tropical Medicine as a practical method of helping his fellow-man, particularly in those countries where poverty is so far below any Western scale. It is this outward-looking spirit that has led him to an important innovation: From 1986 onward, though his Department of International Health and Tropical Medicine, he has hosted an annual lecture at the Royal College of Surgeons in Ireland and has produced as speakers personalities who are as distinguished as they are varied. For an hour each year we can take our hands off the Plough and look at the Stars. And it is a genuine constellation. Intellectual giants are rare in Medicine. Perhaps they are not attracted to its imprecision and are more likely attracted to areas with more tangible and focused problems. The intellectuals we have are often overwhelmed by the ever-more demanding commitments of patient care, teaching, and research.

These talks are brought together for study and reflection. They are the works of men of wide vision. These are the people whose ideas, the most important of all commodities, have influenced the way in which we look at the world.

"Specialisation narrows the mind," said Sir William Olser, the Physician's Physician. Kevin Cahill is not a victim of this. He has always had a breadth of vision and, importantly, a breadth of action to see beyond the confines of medicine to the wider world. To him we owe the opportunity to re-visit these talks given by some of the great minds of our time.

Barry O'Donnell, MCh, FRCSI, FRCS Eng, FRCS ed (ad hom),
President Royal College of Surgeons in Ireland 1999

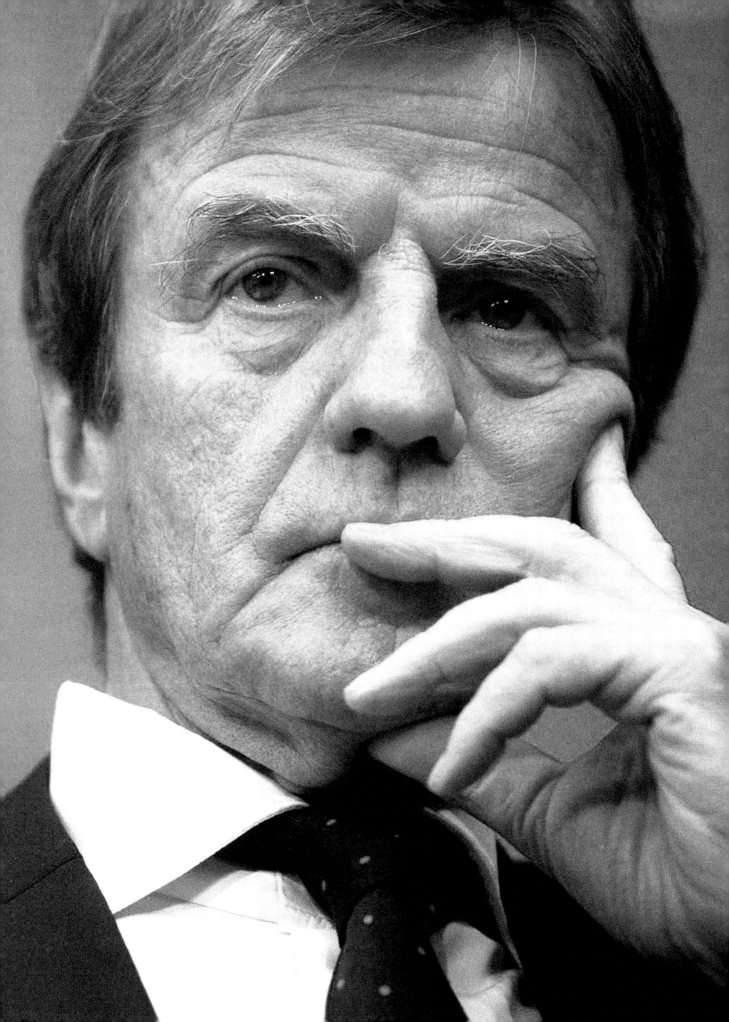

Bernard Kouchner

His Distinguished International Lecture was delivered in the College on October 10, 2006.

The career of Bernard Kouchner incorporates many of the qualities celebrated in a lecture series aimed at expanding the horizons of the medical profession. He received his medical degree from the Université de Paris in 1964, and trained as a gastroenterologist. When the Biafran conflict in Nigeria erupted in 1967, he organized a medical team to provide aid in the war zone. He thought the policy of "medical neutrality" was too confining, believing there was an obligation to forcefully condemn aggressors when necessary. To implement his approach, he founded Médecins Sans Frontières (MSF) or Doctors Without Borders. MSF won the Nobel Peace Prize in 1999. Dr. Kouchner's activism extended both internationally by creating Médecins du Monde (MDM) or Doctors of the World, and nationally by entering French politics. He served as France's first Minister of Humanitarian Affairs, as Minister of Health, and as Foreign Minister. In annual polls in his country over several decades he was selected as the "most admired man in France."

Patients Without Borders
Bernard Kouchner

I. The Birth of a New Conception of Humanitarian Action

I have been for many years involved in fields of work which look different but which in fact converge: humanitarian action, politics and public health. I did develop a famous medical concept, very easy to be stated and difficult to set up: better to prevent than to treat. In many occasions, and in various capacities as volunteer or minister, I have been confronted with the same problem: how to take care of poor people's health, how to let them access to prevention and care?

Biafra

In 1968, I was studying medicine, when the May 1968 movement led by students exploded in France. It was a very restless and creative year. But it was also a very selfish one. Few really cared about "remote" people's misery. Most Westerners were stuck into domestic or personal matters, surely worthy of interest, but with no comparison with the difficulties that were assaulting those whose voice was never heard. France had entered into a new long-lasting period of abundance and mass consumption.

That year, my personal and decisive shock was the war in Biafra. I happened to work there with the International Committee of the Red Cross (ICRC) and face reality. The wounded, the starving children… all of them were denied respect and care because of the supposedly protective Geneva Conventions.

But, we were doctors and we wanted to help different people whose pain and poverty we discovered. The profession had the advantage of being productive across borders and serving a quasi-universal ethical interest. If the sick called on us, we would come, especially if it was forbidden, and sometimes when it was impossible.

A New Concept Of Humanitarian Action: The Responsibility Of Protection

Nationalism was a permanent threat, and indeed often an enemy. In the 1950s and 1960s, the principle that dominated international law was based essentially on the idea of sovereignty of nations. It was, therefore, out of the question to interfere in the internal politics of States which depended only on existing governments, even if these do not emanate from the sovereignty of the people. Any interference generated unanimous criticism from international law specialists from both Western and Eastern countries. But in Biafra we discovered the necessity of free speech and we became illegal to change the law.

The other people's suffering belongs to no one. It is intolerable for governments to consider themselves as the owners of the suffering that they cause. I respect the sovereignty and the legal power of every State. Especially since these guarantee the well being of its people. We only demand that they be exercised in a manner which is more humanitarian and, therefore, more human. I believe that a government that has nothing to hide, could not pull a victim away from the stethoscope of a doctor, or deprive an ordinary man from the advice of a lawyer. Our methods were based on a principle of subsidiarity. It was only after all national resources have been exhausted, that external assistance should be provided. This is what led me, with some of my friends, to create in 1971, Médecins Sans Frontières (Doctors Without Borders), today known as the "French doctors." We were taken for fools for a long time before being awarded the Nobel Peace Prize in 1999.

The "French doctors" are now 15,000 worldwide; they operate in 40 countries, and only for France, its yearly budget amounts to 115.2 million Euros. Unfortunately from one humanitarian crisis to the other, we had to face problem of leadership—inside our group, which like any other, soon developed power struggles in its own ranks, but also of course within the country, the political and social system that we were suddenly involved with, and which in turn had to deal with us. We had to face diversity within our organisation—doctors and nurses coming from various religious, philosophical or political obediences. Our challenge was primarily to confront and convince various ethnic groups which did not share our own conception of medicine and health care. In 1981, I founded *Médecins du Monde* (Doctors of the World), now present in 46 countries.

In 1987, at a "Law and Humanitarian Morality" symposium, I proposed with my friend Mario Bettati, that the French government should adopt the notion of right of interference. And in 1988, United Nations Resolution 43–131 recognised the right of access to victims of natural disasters or similar emergency situations. It was welcomed in Western countries and was not opposed but sometimes worried developing countries that feared colonialism in disguise. Thanks to this new approach, French organisations were able to enter Soviet Armenia in 1988. Six months later, François Mitterrand affirmed: "the obligation of non interference stops exactly where the risk of non assistance begins." In his speech of July 14th 1991, he reminded us that: "France took the initiative for this rather extraordinary right in world history, which is a kind of right of interference inside a country when a section of its population is persecuted." The following year, John Paul II, rallied to the right of interference in order to block the aggressor's hand in Bosnia.

II. State of Affairs

Health Inequalities

Global health is a study in contrasts. The WHO reports that: "while a baby girl born in Japan today can expect to live for about 85 years, a girl born at the same moment in Sierra Leone has a life expectancy of 36 years. The Japanese child will receive vaccinations, adequate nutrition and good schooling. If she becomes a mother she will benefit from high quality maternity care. Growing older, she may eventually develop chronic diseases, but excellent treatment and rehabilitation services will be available; she can expect to receive, on average, medications worth about US $550 per year and much more if needed. One third of global deaths are preventable. One out of every seven children born in a developing country will not survive to age five. There are 42 million people in the world infected with HIV AIDS. There are 12 million AIDS orphans in Africa alone. Malaria kills one million people every year. Tuberculosis is still the greatest killer of adults in the world even though an effective treatment exists. In sub-Saharan Africa, life expectancies have been dropping the last decade – the average life expectancy is now 48 years."

In poor countries, nearly 800 million people do not have enough to eat to stay healthy. Every day, without a guaranteed source of food, they begin their quest. That is their main occupation. Then AIDS arrived, the desert increased, wars multiplied, entire populations were dispersed, and what once was considered worse still is now imaginable. Particularly in Africa, where humanity itself began, the ills of the earth and the sufferance of people are accumulating. The health of the continent in greatest difficulty requires concrete and urgent action. On top of increasingly lethal infectious diseases, famine, or at the very least, nutritional deficiencies and chronic malnutrition is a problem for many, coupled with the increasing emergence of related pathologies. The figures speak for themselves; cases of child mortality, an avoidable problem, can be counted in millions. Diarrhoea, pneumonia, measles, tetanus, meningitis, tuberculosis and malaria subsist when all that is needed is to improve hygiene, to obtain drinking water, to provide proper vaccinations and some basic medicines.

This is all acquired knowledge, and yet these children continue to die, mainly from indifference. Despite the efforts made by some NGOs, despite the basic treatment and vaccination programmes provided by the WHO and UNICEF, despite the WFP and the FAO, children are dying because we provide them with only drops of aid in the desert. We who suffer from plethora and obesity do not know how to share or distribute. We have made the 20th century one of spectacular growth in inequalities of health, living standards, and of knowledge. The relationship of wealth between rich and poor countries has risen from 4 to 80 in 100 years, i.e. 20 times greater. But I am not only speaking of statistics.

Africa is the poorest continent. For example, the total of health expenses per inhabitant is US $3100 (11% PIB) in 2002 in rich countries, whereas it represents only US $81 for (6% PIB) in developing countries. In Africa, the situation is worst with an average of US $37 per inhabitant (5.5% PIB). The number of hospitals beds per 1,000 inhabitants is 7.5 in rich countries, and 1.2 in Africa. The number of doctors is one per 500 inhabitants in rich countries and one per 25,000 in the poorest countries.

Aids: An Example of International Cooperation

AIDS in Africa is a catastrophe of unprecedented proportions. An estimated 4.1 million [3.4 million–6.2 million] became newly infected with HIV and an estimated 2.8 million [2.4 million–3.3 million] lost their lives to AIDS.

Of the estimated 38.6 million [33.4 million–46.0 million] people worldwide living with HIV/AIDS across the world in 2005, 24.5 million [21.6 million–27.4 million] are in Africa. Two million [1.5 million–3.0 million] of them are children younger than 15 years of age.

Are we able to look reality in the face? Can we think of a way of controlling the situation in southern African countries where 30% to 40% of the population is infected? On top of the dramatic consequences of the disease itself that is drastically reducing the life expectancy in these countries, we also have to consider the effects on the entire population in terms of the major economic repercussions, particularly in rural areas: the drop in work capacity, in subsistence crop output, and worsening food shortages. HIV positive women have the difficult choice between breast-feeding, which can transmit HIV to the child, or artificial feeding, which is expensive and presents a danger for the child when water is not drinkable.

The interrelationship of AIDS with other problems of human development has become clearer. It affects societies and economies at various levels, from the family and community to the national and international levels. Current projections suggest that by 2015, in the 60 countries most affected by

AIDS, the total population will be 115 million less than it would be in the absence of AIDS. Africa will account for nearly three-quarters of this difference in 2050, and although life expectancy for the entire continent will have risen to 65.4 years from the current 49.1 years, it will still be almost 12 to 17 years less than life expectancy in other regions of the world.

In Botswana, under-five mortality had been reduced to 62 deaths per thousand live births between 1990 and 1995; today, under-five mortality is approximately 106 deaths per thousand live births. However, the biggest increase in mortality has been among adults aged 20–49, reversing the previous distribution of deaths according to age. Whereas this age group had accounted for only 20% of all deaths between 1985 and 1990, today they account for almost 60%. AIDS strikes down adults in their most economically productive years and removes the very people who could respond to a crisis. Outside of sub-Saharan Africa, in regions with lower HIV prevalence, AIDS has slowed rather than reversed gains in life expectancy.

It is estimated that life expectancy in Cambodia is currently four years lower than it would have been without AIDS. It tends to affect the poor more heavily than other population groups. In Botswana, it is estimated that, on average, every income earner is likely to acquire one additional dependent over the next 10 years due to the epidemic. But families in the poorest quartile will acquire an additional eight people who will become dependent on their income as a result of AIDS. Moreover, a "dramatic" increase in destitute households—those with no income earners—is predicted. Similar findings apply to India, where a review of economic research on AIDS concluded that households belonging to the poor and less educated or unskilled groups, as well as female members of households, face a proportionately greater economic burden due to AIDS. Women in sub-Saharan Africa are infected more often and earlier in their lives than men. Young women aged 15 – 24 are between two and six times as likely to be HIV-positive than men of a similar age.

This evens out in older age groups, but it highlights the vulnerability of young women and girls, and the unequal power relations in many societies. A similar pattern is found in parts of the Caribbean. Although in most parts of the world women live longer than men, AIDS has driven female life expectancy below that of men in four countries: Kenya, Malawi, Zambia and Zimbabwe. Empirical evidence supports the existence of gender differences in mortality. For example, a recent three-year study in Zambia, which involved almost 19,000 people between the ages of 15 and 59, found that 61% of all deaths (i.e. for any cause) occurred among women, and that women on average died at younger ages than did men.

After illness and death itself, the harshest impact on children is the loss of their parents' affection, support and protection. The likelihood of a parent becoming infected if the other parent unknowingly has HIV rises over time. The emotional shock of losing one parent may be inexorably followed by the death of the other. Separation from siblings is frequent as orphans from large families are often sent to live in different households. In addition to the psychological trauma suffered by these children, poverty and social dislocation, as well as stigma and discrimination, may also be added to their woes and in turn increase their vulnerability to HIV. Furthermore, countless children coping with the impact of HIV-related illness on their families become responsible for the care of their siblings and other family members when parents are debilitated by poor health.

Moreover, HIV increases the development of other diseases, in particular tuberculosis, which is rising at a rate of 10% a year. Of the 2 million new cases of tuberculosis diagnosed in Africa in 1999, two-thirds were also infected with HIV. Almost one in every two people with AIDS develops tuberculosis.

Fighting Hunger and Malnutrition in the World

The situation of food in Africa is a chronic catastrophe. Seventeen sub-Saharan African countries are in urgent need of food. The Horn of Africa—Sudan, Somalia and Eritrea—have seen harsh climatic changes, from droughts to excessive rain. When the fragile balance is broken, it results in conflict and the displacement of populations. Africa is home to more than half the world's refugee populations. When stocks run out, prices go up. In southern Africa, Mozambique has also seen worsening food insecurity. Among the forty-seven African countries, only four are considered self-sufficient, despite attempts to develop irrigation and hydraulic equipment. Although cereal production in African has slightly risen from 111.5 tons in 2000 to 116.7 tons in 2001, food dependence has increased, imports are up, and food inequalities are worsening. Southern Africa is the worse affected today with 28 million people facing serious shortages. Africa is the only continent faced with severe increases in food shortages. Over the past twenty years, while the average calorie intake of people in developing countries rose 18%, from 2,150 to 2,520 Kcal/day/pers., in Africa is has fallen by 5% on average.

This average hides the deep and unacceptable disparities, and as food epidemiologists have pointed out, the food situation in Africa is an ongoing tragedy. Because stagnant or disorganised output caused by harsh climatic conditions is worsened by a strong demographic trend that is reducing available resources. We are aware of the consequences, first and foremost, as it affects children. Born by women with deficiencies or anaemia, these children are underweight at birth, a problem that worsens, affecting 30% of children in Africa.

Malnutrition begins in the womb. It worsens at birth by breastfeeding from undernourished women. Overall calorie insufficiency leads to malnutrition, and the cycle continues. Insufficient protein, iodine, iron, and vitamin A intake causes growth and development problems, goitre, anaemia, and seeing problems that number in their millions. Health indicators demonstrate the severity of the problem: life expectancy in sub-Saharan Africa is the lowest in the world at around 50 years, and infant mortality is the highest, especially as that of children under five. These children are malnourished, fragile, lacking in protein and vitamins and are, therefore, exposed to diseases that kill through, brutal and unavoidable epidemics like measles, diarrhoea (800,000 deaths a year), and bronchitis (1.5 million). But these are not the only diseases, which we describe as 'everyday', that are killing children. There are many other diseases that thrive on malnutrition and, in turn, contribute to malnutrition.

Neglected Tropical Diseases

Neglected tropical diseases have afflicted humanity since time immemorial and, in their long histories, have acquired notoriety as disabling and deforming diseases. In the past, their serious impact on health and productivity led to considerable knowledge about the diseases, and effective control tools were developed for many. In addition, as living conditions improved, opportunities for transmission were drastically reduced. As a result, these diseases are now rarely seen in populations that enjoy good access to health services and a reasonable standard of living. Today, neglected tropical diseases are a symptom of poverty and disadvantage. Those most affected are the poorest populations often living in remote, rural areas, urban slums or in conflict zones. With little political voice, neglected tropical diseases have a low profile and status in public health priorities.

Lack of reliable statistics, and unpronounceable names of diseases, have all hampered efforts to bring them out of the shadows. Although medically diverse, neglected tropical diseases share features that allow them to persist in conditions of poverty, where they cluster and frequently overlap. Approximately 1 billion people – one sixth of the world's population – suffer from one or more neglected tropical diseases. Conflict situations or natural disasters aggravate conditions that are conducive to the spread of these diseases. Neglected tropical diseases persist under conditions of poverty and are concentrated almost exclusively in impoverished populations in the developing world. Unsafe water, lack of access to health services, inadequate housing, malnutrition and poor sanitation all increase vulnerability to infection.

Approximately *1 billion people are affected* with one or more neglected tropical diseases. Yet these diseases remain neglected at all levels.

Neglected tropical diseases tend to be hidden below the radar screens of health services and politicians because they afflict populations that are often marginalized, with little political voice. Although frequently causing severe pain and life-long disabilities, these diseases are generally not major killers. Under resource-limited conditions, high mortality diseases such as HIV/AIDS or tuberculosis are prioritized to the detriment of neglected tropical diseases.

Neglected tropical diseases do not travel easily and thus do not pose an immediate threat to Western society. Moreover, they are tied to specific geographical and environmental conditions. The development of new diagnostic tools has been under-funded largely because neglected tropical diseases do not represent a significant market.

Less than 1% of the 1393 new drugs registered during 1975 – 1999 were for tropical diseases. Less than 0.001% of the

US $60 – 70 billion went towards developing new and urgently needed treatments for tropical diseases.

Neglected tropical diseases typically affect the poorest in communities, usually the most marginalized and those least able to demand services. Concentrated almost exclusively in impoverished populations, neglected tropical diseases form a group, with more than 70% of affected countries in low-income or lower middle-income economies.

Many of the neglected tropical diseases can be cured with drugs that cost as little as US $0.02 – $1.50. This figure is cheap for OECD countries with an average GDP per capita of US $28,500 but unaffordable for people earning less than US $1.00 per day. An estimated 1.1 billion people live on less than US $1.00 a day and more than 2.7 billion live on less than US $2.00 a day: they are at higher risk of neglected tropical diseases.

Furthermore, most countries are affected by more than one disease at the same time. International support is essential for scaling up control programmes against neglected tropical diseases. Women and children are more vulnerable.

Women, children and ethnic minorities, as well as those living in remote areas with restricted access to services, are most at risk of infection. In general, women are more exposed to communicable diseases than men – in terms of both morbidity and mortality. Women also face additional barriers to seeking, and often receiving, treatment. The consequences of stigma attached to many neglected tropical diseases are often more severe for women within their families and wider social life. Nearly 70% of all deaths and 75% of all disability-adjusted life years (DALYs) from communicable diseases globally occur in children aged under 14 years. This also applies to neglected tropical diseases as children are much more exposed to infections.

Most neglected tropical diseases cause severe and permanent disabilities but rarely kill. Their low mortality despite high morbidity places them near the bottom of mortality tables and, in the past, they have received low priority. However, the price of neglect is too high; neglected tropical diseases have consequences for affected individuals, families and entire communities in terms of burden of disease, quality of life, loss of productivity and aggravation of poverty. Neglected tropical diseases are a devastating obstacle to human settlement and socioeconomic development of already impoverished countries.

A) Debilitate

Neglected tropical diseases can help guarantee that the next generation remains anchored in poverty. Guinea-worm disease and schistosomiasis have a serious impact on school attendance rates. Sleeping sickness can permanently impair mental function and may cause mental retardation, even in children who are cured. Impaired childhood growth and cognitive development are associated with schistosomiasis and soil-transmitted helminthiasis.

B) Deform

Deformities associated with neglected tropical diseases such as leprosy, leishmaniasis and lymphatic filariasis can become so severe that patients are banished from their communities as well as the work force. These are the severely enlarged limbs of elephantiasis, the faces eroded by mucocutaneous leishmaniasis or leprosy, and the limbs of small children that are amputated to save their lives from aggressive Buruli ulcer infection.

C) Blind

Occurring as it does in rural areas, blindness caused by onchocerciasis and trachoma can jeopardize food security and cause dramatic changes in patterns of land use. On the river Koni, in the Bani basin of Mali, a staff member spent the morning with a blind couple who had been brought to a field by a child and who spent the long day slowly picking out the unwanted grass from between the millet, differentiating the two by the feel of their leaves. These images, multiplied by a hundred thousand, are the human face of onchocerciasis.

D) Kill

Untreated, human African trypanosomiasis (sleeping sickness) and leishmaniasis are killers. Sleeping sickness invariably progresses to body wasting, somnolence, coma and death. Visceral leishmaniasis damages the internal organs such as liver, spleen and bone marrow. Left untreated, it is usually fatal within two years. Most neglected tropical diseases can be prevented and even eliminated if affected communities have timely access to existing effective tools. The challenge at hand is to scale up coverage and access to these tools on a proactive, preventive basis.

High pay-off, low-cost tools in several cases, population-wide interventions, such as vector control and mass drug administration, are powerful enough to interrupt transmission. For most neglected tropical diseases, safe, effective and low-cost technologies are currently available. A dramatic reduction in communicable diseases could be achieved at the minimal cost of about US $0.40 per person per year. Community or school-based deworming through mass drug administration is another highly cost-effective intervention at US $6–33 per DALY gained.

An Integrated Approach To Vanquishing Diseases

An integrated framework to tackle multiple diseases affecting the same communities needs to be urgently adopted. This would combine vector control, heavily reliant on judicious use of pesticides, and preventive chemotherapy to all populations at risk of infection. Core activities such as service delivery, logistics, and monitoring and surveillance can be pooled for use across various diseases, with evident savings and efficiencies.

Feasible in resource-poor settings control of many neglected tropical diseases relies on simple interventions that can be carried out by non-specialists, for example schoolteachers, village heads and local volunteers.

Local Ownership

Neglected tropical diseases have the advantage of being a high priority for affected communities. This creates an opportunity for a head-start by relying on principles of local ownership, health education and community-based preventive action. In some parts of the world, interventions that produce immediate results—pain relief, elimination of household insects, expulsion of intestinal worms—increase acceptance of control programmes in affected communities and stimulate local demand. Marketing Discriminatory attitudes and prejudices contribute to the spread of neglected tropical diseases and worsen their impact on those affected.

Mass Public Awareness Campaign for Eliminating Stigma Attached to Leprosy

For a long time, leprosy was considered shameful and people hid their symptoms for fear of ostracism despite free and effective multidrug therapy. The disease was therefore detected only at a late stage after irreversible disabilities had set it. In 1990, one Ministry of Health, assisted by international support, launched a powerful and broad-based advertising campaign to change the public image of leprosy. By portraying leprosy as just another treatable disease, the campaign hoped to encourage people with suspicious lesions to come forward for early diagnosis and cure free of charge.

The campaign virtually eliminated the stigma attached to leprosy. The image of leprosy has moved from one of fear and loathing to one of hope and cure. Since the start of the campaign, more than 20,000 patients have been detected and treated. In less than a year, case detection had increased by 150%. In the year before the campaign, only 9% of new cases were self-reported; that figure rose to 50% by 1991 and has remained high in subsequent years. Leprosy has been eliminated at a national level since 1996. In 1995, the national prevalence rate dropped below 1 per 10,000 population. Leprosy has been eliminated in Sri Lanka since 1996. Since 2002, leprosy control activities are now fully integrated into general health services to maintain the country's triumph over leprosy.

Patients Without Borders

If we believe that the health of people is a universal good, capable of transcending cultures, religions, and beliefs, if we all aspire to this around the world, we need to define a level of health that is compatible with life and not survival. Let us not take account of the naïve concepts of the WHO, *the complete state of physical and mental well-being.* No one aware of the state of the world we live in could accept such a mechanistic definition, except for rare moments of love-making ecstasy.

As G. Canguilhem pointed out (*Le normal et le pathologique*), health is not the absence of disease, but an ability to withstand one's environment. Withstanding all these ills is to refuse the factors that create them. What are the choices we have? Refusal. Refusal of fatalism, barbarity and dictatorship, refusal of the confiscation of goods, technology, knowledge and power. The struggle against illiteracy, and the promotion of the place of women in schools and in decisive positions are concrete actions whose positive effects are largely valued and recognised.

These actions are a primary necessity, but this alone is not enough. The world's organisation should be built on respect for the rights of its inhabitants. A world in which the inevitability of massive and recurrent famine would not exist. Our planet can feed 6 billion humans beings today and 10 billion tomorrow. We only need to make a choice: a choice to share and to intervene, a choice to respect the rights of life.

The French health monitoring system analyses and surveys the various populations of the world and is able to identify the risks and anticipate health and human catastrophes. Warning is therefore possible. Must we, and can we, let these hungry people die? The choice of society is a political choice that we have to accept responsibility for. Therein lies the ability to act. The responsibility of all those who share the immense privilege of living in a democracy is directly involved.

We have to fight against our fears that generate useless, disproportionate, harmful withdrawal. Of course every victim has the right to our compassion. And they should be counted one by one. But how to differentiate with such a feeling of indifference? The 600 dead from SARS (severe acute respiratory syndrome) in Asia last spring shook the world with a frightening and unprecedented media frenzy, while several hundreds of thousands of children died in silence and indifference from curable diseases. A cliché, some will say, but this is the forgotten reality of exclusion. Our fears are the instruments that orientate our policies, be they health or otherwise.

Malades Sans Frontiers (Patients Without Borders) is not a slogan, but a clearly visible reality. We know what has to be done: a worldwide health insurance system. By starting small, I find myself in the same situation as when we began Médecins Sans Frontières (MSF). The movement is taking form; as we speak a worldwide tax, a universal income. I had the proposed, the "Tobin tax," voted at the European Parliament with Daniel Cohn-Bendit in 1994; I remain a fervent defender of it: taxation of capital flows, in one form or another. We would start with volunteer banks, as we did for ethical fundraising. Those who speak of a universal tax say it is quite possible, and that a very small percentage would suffice. I am not claiming it would be financially easy, nor would it be simple in terms of infrastructure, but it is a fight we are winning. It is a trend that is catching on.

The word 'globalisation' cannot be used to denote the negative alone. This will change. By creating MSF, people took us for medical hippies. But this too changed. I feel comfortable in this movement, in the need to organise globalisation. The solutions put forward by the anti-globalisation movement are not always pertinent. But their indignation, their demands, and the way they present their arguments—except the extreme violent— I understand and approve. France was the precursor to this whole movement with *French Doctors*. They were not the representatives of the French foreign ministry any more than they were from civil society. They came from an ideal France.

The power of this movement was underestimated at first. What did we say? However poor, dirty, or uncultivated, the human being in front of us—and God knows I am not being pejorative—this was a sick person and we had to provide treatment. And then, before long, we said, "This is our sick person, beyond borders." We provided medicine. It was a fine movement, but it very quickly became insufficient.

Globalisation will not only signify grand but empty gatherings, nor a worldwide love of football. Tomorrow we will create minimum social protection for the poor of the world: "Malades sans frontiers."

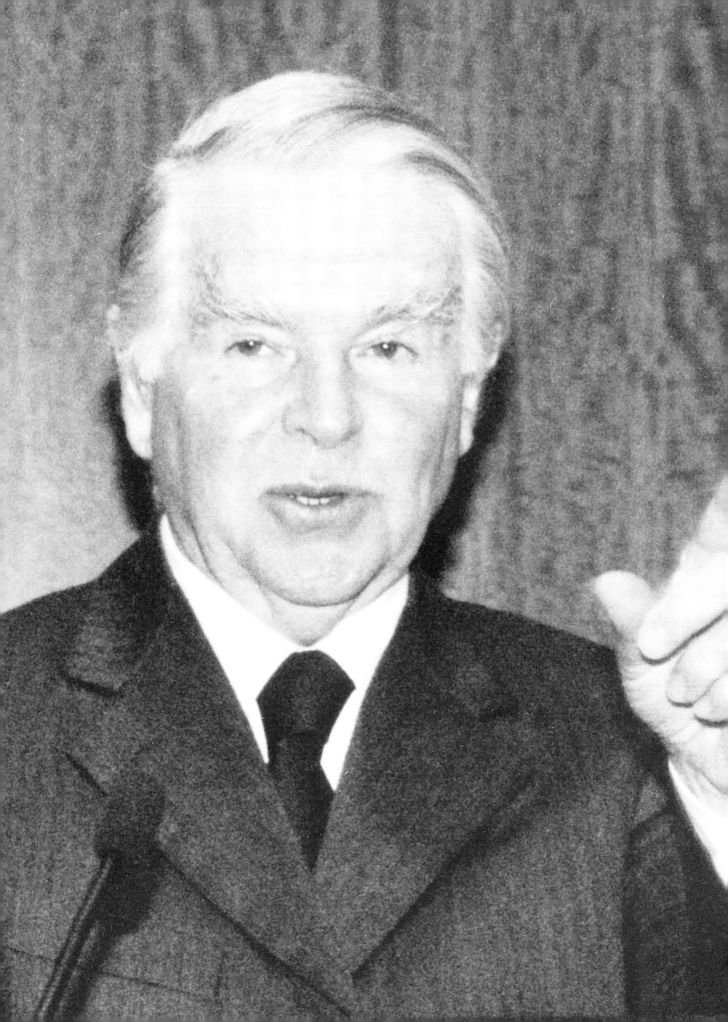

Kevin M. Cahill M.D.

His Distinguished International Lectures were delivered in the College on February 6, 2006 and June 25, 1998.

Kevin M. Cahill M.D. was the first Professor and Chairman of the Department of Tropical Medicine at the Royal College of Surgeons. He, and his late wife, Kate, sponsored the Distinguished International Lecture Series that is presented in this book. His medical career has evolved from that of a clinician to one embracing the complexities of international humanitarian relief assistance. He has worked in disaster areas, conflict zones, and refugee camps in over 70 countries. He has served as the Chief Advisor in Humanitarian and Public Health for three Presidents of the United Nations.
He has received numerous academic and diplomatic awards. The first Lecture was delivered when the College appointed him to a newly created Professorship in International Humanitarian Affairs; a decade earlier he delivered the lecture from which the first edition of this book drew its subtitle.

A Bud of Thought That Wants to Be a Rose
Kevin M. Cahill, M.D.

The ancient arts of healing have drawn upon many disciplines to create an incredibly rich history, possibly the most noble record of human endeavor. Those of us privileged to have the practice of medicine as a "way of life" may be better armed than any other profession to help a rapidly changing world order avoid utter collapse. My talk this evening details my own evolution into fields where dreams and reality coalesced; as the Nicaraguan poet, Rubén Darío once wrote, different phases of my career have represented "a bud of thought that wants to be a rose." The philosophy of the Royal College of Surgeons in Ireland provided, I believe, the solid foundation needed for both personal and institutional transitions that embrace activities once thought to be the domain of only statesmen and security analysts.

The Department of Tropical Medicine was officially begun at the RCSI in 1969. Since a history of its activities has been published, I will not reiterate details here except to emphasize the academic undertakings that fostered new initiatives and encouraged an "open door" approach to new challenges.

The methodology of public health was adapted to serve the needs of diplomacy; our profession's focus on early detection, rapid assessment, diagnosis and appropriate therapy offered a model for unraveling the causes of conflicts, and even discovering those elusive paths to healing the wounds and scars of traumatized populations. This was the basis for my book, *Preventive Diplomacy: Stopping Wars Before They Start,* and numerous nations have now adopted formal policies seeking alternatives to the recurrent, failed approaches of the past, ones emphasizing only revenge, military reactions, retribution, sanctions, and the endless games of power politics.

All around the globe medical and health personnel enjoy an enormous untapped reservoir of respect and credibility. They are in a unique position to see, and interpret, the realities and wonders of life and, if they act with decency and dignity, health professionals are accepted by people of all races, creeds and political beliefs. Capitalizing on this provides an "open door," and that is what this Distinguished Lecture promotes – accepting the challenge of expanding the horizons of medicine, breaking artificial barriers so that our profession can help meet new threats to an old world order.

These threats are not merely drug resistant and emerging infections, epidemics or environmental disasters. They include natural and man-made disasters, and terrorist activity, requiring innovative responses that reflect a more deep understanding of other's behaviors. Furthermore, as we retaliate against evil foes, we must be careful to not destroy those precious civil liberties that are the foundation of our own societies. As I accept my second Professorship at the RCSI, one in International Humanitarian Affairs, I am offered a far broader and more complex canvas.

This Distinguished Lecture records the evolution of a tropicalist, a journey from a physician's traditional focus on the signs and symptoms of disease, devising appropriate therapy to cure individual patients, on to a career handling complex humanitarian crises with responsibility for sheltering, feeding, securing, triaging, treating, and even educating hundreds of thousands of vulnerable people, mostly women and children, in make-shift refugee camps, and then, later, to the medical and public health aspects of counterterrorism.

Humanitarian Assistance

"Humanitarian crises" are rarely the result of just a failure of the humanitarian system. Solutions, therefore, will not be found by merely addressing unmet humanitarian needs. My experiences in refugee camps—where traumatized and displaced persons who had fled conflicts and often lost everything—raised many questions regarding our almost predictable patterns of assistance based on a Western clinical approach. Slowly, but steadily, such observations led me, more and more, deeply into unchartered seas. From both a philosophic and professional point of view, I came to resent those who believed a physician should confine himself solely to the socially accepted parameters of clinical medicine. I began to write books and articles asserting that medical life, especially in conflict zones, and where states and societies were collapsing, actually offered an almost unique vantage point from which one could experience, come to understand, and try to describe a very sad world we rarely —and barely—knew. Maybe, just maybe, it might provide the basis for new initiatives, modest, humble but inherently noble actions, that would allow comprehensive contact with oppressed and forgotten peoples who survived almost without hope.

There are many factors that influence complex humanitarian crises; the medical, demographic, epidemiological, and logistical ones are easily measured, and effective responses can usually be formulated. Yet it is those less definable, more subjective, forces that so often determine the course of events. As in human relations, it is usually the subtle, but utterly essential, influences of natural empathy and understanding; a respect for the diversity of humanity; an appreciation of others' values and customs; a willingness to cooperate, and share; the courage to give, to accept, to understand, and even embrace other's concerns, that most often provide the critical defining balance between success and failure in refugee settings.

One of the most serious problems when I began working in humanitarian crises in the early 1960's was the lack of a common vocabulary, of almost any widely accepted standards, or academically solid training. Academic interest in granting diplomas or degrees to field workers was non-existent. We began–first here at the RCSI–a postgraduate program, the International Diploma in Humanitarian Assistance (IDHA). It now has over 2,300 graduates from 133 nations, and serves every United Nations agency, numerous international and local non-governmental organizations (NGOs), as well as military, missionary, medical, legal, and other personnel representing all the many disciplines that contribute in humanitarian crises. By joining academia (with its analytical and research capacity) and relief workers (with their unique field experience in disasters) a profession is beginning to develop from the confusion that was typical decades ago. The IDHA has provided a critical foundation for that emerging profession.

Professionals in humanitarian assistance must approach those in pain in a nonjudgmental manner. They learn to leave behind their pride, and their preconceptions, and to sublimate their own interests and agendas in an act of solidarity with refugees and displaced persons. One learns to tread softly, to offer change with great care. One quickly finds that existing customs and practice in any community, even in the chaos of refugee camp, must not be altered without consultation and deliberation. The ways of a people, sometimes quite incomprehensible to one trained in a Western scientific system, are ultimately that group's own precious heritage and protection. Attempts to introduce new methods, and replace time-worn approaches can be devastating, especially in times of crisis, when the failure of their society makes people extremely vulnerable, while also being completely dependent on strangers for the essentials of life.

In humanitarian crises, one also struggles with the dark and tangled roots of hatred and incipient revenge, passions that, maybe understandably, flourish and explode among the dispossessed in settings of loss and unrelenting misery. One quickly becomes aware that there are no simple answers in such situations. Solutions, when they can be constructed, draw on many, many skills. It was essential to extend the professional standards that prevailed in clinical tropical medicine to the less-disciplined field of humanitarian affairs, and that is what has been done at the RCSI. Disaster management is an evolving science, embracing every stage from prevention and preparedness, through cluster assignments to the final phases of reconstruction and development.

When I was young, and very innocent, I thought I was inordinately important as a medical doctor in a refugee camp. But it did not take long to look around and realize, with growing humility, that those in charge of water or food or shelter or security or sanitation or education were essential partners. It certainly did not take long to realize that no one could accomplish very much working alone. I came to understand that if there was to be any progress in restoring a semblance of stability for those who had lost almost everything, we had to overcome our own restrictive professional barriers.

One had to develop a radically different perspective regarding those treasured academic distinctions we had been taught were so important during medical training. One had to learn not to be afraid to venture afield as circumstances demanded.

Diplomas and degrees can easily become artificial boxes that prevent flexibility. In providing humanitarian assistance, flexibility is an indispensable and absolute necessity.

For decades, I have been privileged to work in remote areas among people far removed from the effects—good and bad—of modernity. The more I traveled, and read, and participated in the daily lives of isolated tribes the more convinced I was that the richness of humanity lay in its incredible diversity. I do not share the belief that there is only one right way—whether that is how to rule, or how to worship, or court a mate, or establish a family, or express love, or even how to die. Any diminution in that diversity diminishes all of us. Attempts to homogenize the world, to impose uniform standards of behavior, to stifle differences of opinion and style, to impose restrictions on customs and practices because they are different from our own are regressive, usually destructive, acts. The biologic world thrives in its complexity, and artistic creativity flourishes best when there are multiple varying stimuli.

In one of his memorable books, Conor Cruise O'Brien reminded us that, ultimately, ideas matter most. These new ideas, this new dimension of International Humanitarian Affairs now in RCSI's mandate, provides a broader definition of medicine's boundaries, one that may allow us to find new ways of understanding the roots of evil, why they flourish, and how we must address them.

Counterterrorism

I did not choose my next "career," but in the post 9/11 world of America, it became clear there was a major need for medical expertise in counterterrorism. The lessons of humanitarian assistance were magnified many fold when I was thrust into the dark world of counterterrorism, including advising on biological agents that had become deadly terrorist's tools.

When I lived in the Middle East more than four decades ago I had diagnosed many patients with anthrax; one learned to recognize the classical clinical picture of an eschar or severe pulmonary disease; one learned how to isolate the etiologic bacteria, and prescribe appropriate therapy. Now I had to learn how terrorists could weaponize anthrax into powder form so that it could be silently disseminated across a nation. We had to find ways to detect and decontaminate, and, maybe most importantly, to try to comprehend the motivations of those who use bioterrorist weapons. Society has every right to protect itself against terrorists, and I learned much from professional colleagues in the intelligence and security communities. These efforts were usually in response to very real and potential attacks, but their reactions rarely probed deeply, as physicians are trained to do, into the underlying causes.

The 2001 bioterrorist attacks with anthrax in America not only killed innocent victims but resulted in the closing of the United States Supreme Court, the House of Representatives and several of the major television networks. These new and anonymous attacks caused panic in security forces across the country. Ignorance and fear paralyzed a nation. When I was asked to become the Chief Medical Advisor for Counterterrorism for the New York Police Department (NYPD), police officers bluntly told me they would not hesitate to run down a dark alley shooting – and being shot at – by a thief. But they would refuse to go into a potentially contaminated building or subway station, concerned – and confused – about how they might bring fatal diseases home to their families in suburbia. An intensive educational program was begun, in which I learned as much about the minds of the police – and terrorists – as they learned from me.

Terrorism emerges from blind hatred of an other, and that in turn is the product of three factors: fear, rage and incomprehension.

Fear of what the other might do to you, rage at what you believe the other has done to you, and incomprehension about who or what the other really is—these three elements fuse together in igniting the deadly combustion that kills and destroys people whose only sin is that they feel none of these things themselves.

If terrorism is to be tackled and ended, we will have to deal with each of these three factors by attacking the ignorance that sustains them. We will have to know each other better, learn to see ourselves as others see us, learn to recognize hatred and deal with its causes, learn to dispel fear, and, above all, just learn more about each other. In one sense, the terrorists of 2001 were attacking the globalization of the human imagination—the godless, materialist, promiscuous culture of the dominant West, embodied in a globalization from which people like them felt excluded. Certainly those who celebrated their acts did so from a sense of exclusion. If we speak of the human imagination today, we need to ask what leads surprisingly large numbers of young people to follow the desperate course set for them by fanatics and ideologues. A sense of oppression, of exclusion, of marginalization, gives rise to extremism.

A half century ago, in 1962, the now all-but-forgotten UN Secretary General U Thant warned that an explosion of violence could occur as a result of the sense of injustice felt by those living in poverty and despair in a world of plenty. Some 2,600 people died in New York's World Trade Center on 9/11/2001. But some 26,000 people also died around the world on that same day – from starvation, unclean water and preventable diseases. We cannot afford to exclude them from our global imagination. Those who suffer, and are rejected, are the predictable perpetrators of future terrorist attacks, and no amount of counterintelligence or preemptive attacks will stamp out these huge populations. If health workers have the skills to heal individuals, as well as the tools to stop epidemics and even eliminate diseases from the face of the earth, then we should not–in fact we cannot–absent ourselves from this new war on terrorism, a war with no apparent end and few definable borders. New solutions are obviously needed, and they may lie unappreciated in the rich traditions of our medical profession.

For me the winds of globalization must blow both ways. The UNESCO Charter memorably tells us that "as war begins in the minds of men, it is in the minds of men that the foundations of peace must be constructed." This is true not just for war and peace, but in every aspect of human life and society for which lasting foundations must be constructed in the mind. As the acolytes of Osama bin Laden, or the young foot soldiers of the Taliban, have taught us, the globe will always have more than a single mind. And that is why cultural diversity is so essential in our shrinking globe. For without a multiplicity of cultures, we cannot realize how peoples of other races, religions or languages share the same dreams; the same hopes. Without a heterogeneous human imagination, we cannot understand the myriad manifestations of the human condition, nor fully appreciate the universality of human aims and aspirations.

I have perhaps taken too long in tackling the themes I raised at the beginning of this lecture. So let me pull the threads together. In much of the world there exist societies whose richness lies in their soul and not in their soil, whose past may offer more wealth than their present, whose imagination is more valuable than their technology. Recognizing that this might be the case, and affirming that the imagination is as central to humanity's sense of its own worth as the ability to eat and drink and sleep under a roof, is part of the challenge before the world today. The only way to ensure that this challenge is met is to preserve cultural and imaginative freedom in all societies, to guarantee that individual voices find expression, that all ideas and forms of art are enabled to flourish and contend for their place in the sun. We have heard in the past that the world must be made safe for democracy. That goal is increasingly being realized in many parts of the world, an often incremental process that is not dramatic except in retrospect. More human rights, gender equality, and other democratic freedoms are now taken for granted in societies where they would have been inconceivable a generation ago. Future progress may seem to some too slow, but the movement forward seems, at least to me, inevitable. It is now time for all of us to work to make the world safe for diversity.

There are obvious different approaches in the search for safety and peace in a world of diversity. Individuals, for example, usually enjoy freedom of choice and expression, though in politically volatile areas expressions must be discreet and respectful of foreign mores. On the other hand, especially in conflict or post-conflict zones, where tensions are high, organizations, such as international humanitarian agencies and academic institutions, must strive to find a balance where they both uphold their ethical traditions while maintaining a "neutral space," in which they can deliver services as impartially as possible. That balance can sometimes be confused by outspoken individuals perceived to articulate a position for an entire organization. It is critical that such errors be avoided by proper leadership, and, if they do occur, are corrected promptly and transparently.

I would like to conclude with several related observations for my fellow medical colleagues. The constant challenges, the humbling failures, the unreasonable demands, the slings and arrows of clinical life, participating in the joys and sorrows of birth and pain, healing and death, are our daily privileges. How we can translate this experience to disaster management and counterterrorism, to diplomacy and politics, has long obsessed me.

I have been caught behind the lines in too many armed conflicts, and seen senseless slaughter from the Middle East to Managua, and all across the scarred landscape of Africa. Somehow, in the twisted wreckage of war, and in the squalor of refugee camps, the beauty of humanity prevailed for me. If you too can find this eternal radiance in life, and look around a world in desperate need of your help, then have the courage to step out of the box.

Do not be frightened by the unknown, or shy away from challenges that were not part of your training, for you will quickly realize that others on the scene have no greater capacity, and, in fact, have usually had a much more narrow educational base. Do not place false restrictions on, or in any way limit, your options. If you can offer the ethos of our profession to a world starved for order and competency, social justice and the rights of the frail and oppressed – and that is what the Hippocratic oath encourages you to do – then, when opportunity presents, and it will in the most unexpected and exciting ways, do not let it escape. There are many hidden buds of thought that can blossom into roses, and we're only on this earth once. There is an overdue opportunity to make a difference.

Health and Foreign Policy
Kevin M. Cahill, M.D.

The foreign policy of any nation reflects its fears and dreams as well as its own particular political and economic interests. In the Cold War era, convinced that its national security was under constant mortal threat, the United States allowed the element of fear to become a dominant influence. Its overseas agenda failed to appreciate that the growing disparities between rich and poor, hungry and nourished, free and oppressed had become the driving forces in conflicts around the world. During the same period the global landscape was changing, challenging traditional concepts of sovereignty, borders and nationalism.

Particularly in Africa, Central America, the Balkans, and in parts of the former Soviet Union, and Afghanistan, a form of perpetual war, based on ethnic factors and parochial greed, replaced classic warfare between states. These battles were fought with a level of brutality and cruelty that was without precedent, and many current conflicts take place without even recognized governments to deal with. Accepted standards of medical neutrality are rarely recognized, or even understood, by combatants. International humanitarian law, the rules of war, and the Geneva conventions are as unknown as they are unenforceable in most conflicts today. On my last trip to Somalia 12-year-old children with AK-47s were the law at most road blocks.

We must, obviously, devise new methods to deal more effectively with these difficult realities. All nations, particularly the powerful and rich, must learn that they can afford to be compassionate as well as strong, and by emphasizing health and humanitarian assistance could fashion a foreign policy capable of rekindling a fraternal spirit that is now being strangled, at home and abroad, by cynicism, selfishness and false isolationism.

Think for a moment—and, if you do, you will be among the minuscule number who seem to be thinking about such matters of recent crises that demonstrate why health issues should be absolutely central in every nation's foreign policy. Health issues are usually considered—if they are considered at all—as peripheral concerns by those who formulate and implement our overseas agendas. Yet I offer the following examples:

1) When Ebola breaks out in the Congo or plague erupts in India, the old logic of quarantine is irrelevant. The speed of travel and the mass movement of people have destroyed any assurance of isolation of, or protection against, the spread of deadly diseases. Epidemics can threaten a nation's basic security as surely as nuclear weapons, yet the imbalance in government spending is appalling. For example, in the 1997 American Foreign Aid Bill, twenty times more dollars were allocated for military aid to other nations than were set aside for all foreign disaster assistance.

2) Consider the impact of HIV infection and AIDS in Africa. Are these purely medical concerns? The Washington Post recently wrote an editorial about a study on my desk, which

shows that over 50% of the armed forces in seven African nations are HIV positive. This is not a surprising figure when you consider that soldiers are young, relatively wealthy, mobile, and have a tradition of imposing their will along the highways and chaotic areas that characterize so much of turbulent Africa. But if you simultaneously consider that the very stability of most African states is predicated, for better or worse, on the military, then you must conclude that the fundamental foundation of these nations is fragile indeed, resting on a group of very sick people with a predictable and very short life-expectancy, who hold power in areas where the diagnosis of, and medications for, AIDS are simply not available. The annual average health budget in many poor African countries is between $5 and $10 per capita, while the cost for antiviral drugs alone is approximately $15,000 per person per year.

3) To even further complicate the African AIDS disaster and to emphasize the diplomatic implications of health issues, it should be noted that no pre-employment HIV tests are required when the United Nations deploys armed divisions from endemic zones to be part of their 'Blue Beret' forces. Therefore, troops dedicated to peacekeeping are undoubtedly simultaneously contributing to the dissemination of fatal infections.

4) Possibly the best case study for demonstrating the relationship between health and foreign policy is the global land mine crisis. There are 100 million mines buried in over 60 countries, the lethal residue of almost forgotten wars. Innocent victims, most often women and children, are being blown up decades after the end of conflicts due to these horrific hidden weapons. Land mine injuries are clearly a topic with multiple medical implications, and one could, as a physician,

focus merely on the tragic details of traumatic injuries, the infectious complications of shrapnel wounds, the problems of developing rehabilitation programs in war zones, the costly burden of extensive surgery and blood transfusions on health budgets in tropical areas, or on the diversionary impact of such therapeutic procedures on basic immunization, prenatal, nutritional and other public health programs.

In 1995 I described the situation I knew well in a mine infested area of Northern Somalia: 'In the fertile grazing grounds of Somaliland mothers now tie toddlers to trees so that the young children cannot crawl, innocently but dangerously, out among the more than one million mines that have been haphazardly laid there over the last decade. Camels, and the youngsters and adolescents who tend them, are less fortunate, since to survive in the Somali savannah, animals must endlessly search for water and nourishment. The fields are littered with camel carcasses, and stone mounds mark the graves of herders. The towns are crowded with amputees. Mine injuries have become one of the major health hazards in that sad country, reaching epidemic proportions in the north.' Similar scenes characterize significant portions of countries in an alphabetical line from Angola and Afghanistan, to Cambodia, the Sudan and on to the former Yugoslavia.

I first became interested in land mine victims in the 1980s when I saw the same faces in the same Nicaraguan hospital beds, month after month, year after year, during the Contra-Sandinista war. I tried to adapt an inexpensive Indian prosthesis – the Jaipur Foot – to the Nicaraguan needs. For a number of almost predictable reasons, my effort largely failed and I analyzed that failure in a book entitled *Clearing the Fields: Solutions to the Land Mine Crisis.*

When I developed a new amputee program in Hargeisa,

Northern Somalia, I tried to avoid the errors made in Nicaragua. I had kept a research team in Somalia for 30 consecutive years, knew the people and terrain well, and much of my own epidemiologic writing was based on field work in the Horn of Africa. During the early 1990s, as Somalia disintegrated as a nation, a grant was secured from the African Development Bank to see whether one could establish a viable rehabilitation project in a war zone where there were no doctors, no hospitals, no government, no police, no electricity – in short there was total and utter anarchy.

Within five months, using only amputees to construct a modest medical facility, and importing Jaipur feet and material for limbs over a very dangerous land route from Djibouti, the rehabilitation project was fully functioning, with newly trained technicians fitting over 100 amputees per month with artificial limbs. We were able to establish and preserve the program solely because the clan system, and the influence of elders and sheikhs, protected the rehabilitation compound. We kept the technology as simple and the costs as low as possible. Our Somali below-the-knee prostheses cost $18, and patients received a one-day rehabilitation program. In comparison, a below-the-knee prosthesis in New York costs over $4,000, and most patients undergo a three-month rehabilitation and training regimen. Few public health programs are as visibly successful as suddenly seeing hundreds of legless men, women and children walking around town. The Somali project has now been replicated in war-destroyed areas of Angola, Mozambique and Afghanistan.

Soldiers, politicians, diplomats, humanitarian and human rights activists can all approach the global land mine crisis from differing vantage points, and all bring their own valuable perceptions and prejudices. One could focus, for example, on the economic burden, especially in impoverished nations, of the terrible waste of arable lands abandoned because of the danger of mines, or reflect on the profound psychological scars that are the inevitable end result of surviving with the constant threat of explosions. But one does not cease to be a citizen merely because one uses a stethoscope and it is, as a physician/citizen, that one may be able to offer the most authoritative insights to the complex challenge of land mines in foreign policy.

The physician who is able to transcend his own professional agenda, and be sensitive to problems beyond the traditional concerns of medicine, may have a unique contribution to make. The physician brings to the diplomatic table an unusual credibility and acceptability; in clinical medicine, there is a strength that flows from personal service and an authority that derives directly from having cared for the very real problems of individual victims.

The relationship of health and foreign policy is not a theoretical exercise. Today, many, if not most foreign interventions by developed nations are now predicated, or at least defended, on humanitarian bases—starving Somalis, homeless Kurds, dead Rwandans. Yet, in my experience, few political or diplomatic leaders understand the health and humanitarian issues they so readily invoke, and they rarely involve health or humanitarian workers in developing or implementing the policies that guide its national actions overseas. It is certainly true that this failure can be the fault of the health professions.

At the time of the Nicaraguan war, in the *Journal of Public Health Policy*, I noted: "The current American policy toward Nicaragua poses a fundamental challenge to those who consider themselves the leaders of our public health. Those who absent themselves from the present national debate, who seek anonymity in silence, who fear to venture forth from the safe harbors and shoals of academia, will have sacrificed a rare opportunity as professionals and as citizens."

Too rarely have health professionals been willing to venture into the rough-and-tumble world of public life where the protective coat of specialized knowledge has, sadly, been more of a shield than a sword. Albert Einstein once indicted his professional colleagues thus: "Intellectuals," he said, "are cowards, even more than most people. They have failed miserably when called on to fight for dangerous convictions. Anyone who seeks to affect the course of events must exert direct influence on men and their activities." In bringing some balance to what I believe is a serious distortion of America's heritage, a foreign policy that violates almost every principle we were once taught to treasure, health workers may be an untapped resource.

Health professionals are among the most educated and, occasionally, the most respected members of a community. Yet, except when an issue impinges on their particular interest, their impact on government policy is minuscule. A physician may have the most privileged role, especially in societies where there are multiple reasons for suspicion or cynicism or even hatred. By a mutual sharing, the good physician becomes part of the body and soul of the person he serves. If that trust and confidence are not abused, and if, with warmth and humility and competency, the doctor proves his worth over time, the bond becomes as durable as love. When people and nations can agree on little else, those common bonds may become the bridge back to understanding and peace. There is certainly no reason not to utilize this bridge, especially in light of the dismal record of standard diplomacy.

I extended this argument in a subsequent book, *A Framework for Survival*. By building on common objectives and universally accepted values, by defining the core needs of all human beings and proposing ways to satisfy those needs, we may be able to create a better framework for survival in a new century. Focusing on health, human rights and humanitarian assistance offers an innovative approach to foreign policy that may be more effective in many cases than the conventional military, economic, and geopolitical "solutions" that have so often been so flawed. Time is not on the side of those who believe we can maintain the status quo, that we can continue to confront reality with old rhetoric and allow the past to happen over and over again.

With today's communications, it is impossible to hide from distant catastrophes. Bloated bellies and destroyed societies are no longer only sad stories to be debated by statesmen far removed in time and space from the carnage. Now the images are on our television screens; they are a major force in our own and our children's continuous education. Unless we intend to give up being human, we can no longer feel warm and secure in our homes while disasters swirl through the cold world outside.

The fact that we know, instantly and vividly, that terrible wrongs are occurring creates a moral and legal burden that did not weigh on previous generations. No amount of sophistry can ever again humanize the horrors of war or the waste of innocent lives into dull statistics that soften the harsh fact that it is real people who suffer and die. We cannot simply talk about problems, deceiving ourselves that words—even heartfelt concerns—can substitute for corrective actions and compassionate deeds.

I have had the good fortune to work as a physician for four decades in troubled areas of Africa, Latin America, and Asia. I have shared in the human catastrophes that are an inevitable part of conflicts, and in the tragedies that follow earthquakes and famines, droughts and floods. I learned the humbling lessons of Third World medicine, that politics and prejudice, racism and religion, weather and witchcraft, corruption and incompetence, were as much a part of most nations' health problems as the easily definable diseases we were taught in medical school. I also saw firsthand that economic embargoes are not abstractions, the antiseptic instruments of power politics. They are anesthesia supplies that do not come, respirators that cannot be repaired, and people who needlessly die.

These experiences convinced me that those health care workers who have intimate contact with the suffering of the masses, as well as unusual access to foreign leaders, could contribute to the solution of crises and conflicts in ways impossible for politicians, soldiers, and even diplomats. Humanitarian actions can open doors to negotiated settlements; even in the midst of violence, they can create corridors of understanding that eventually become permanent bridges to peace.

However, even opening doors, or establishing corridors, may have little impact on the prevention or resolution of conflicts. To change the perceptions of responsibility, the traditional prerogatives of actors in a political process, is not easy, and comes slowly. Politicians usually consider health workers as very nice do-gooders who are presumed to be too innocent to understand the harsh realities of diplomatic decision making. Health workers are usually used to justify interventions, to assist in relief efforts, particularly if the media can record a nation's compassion, and then they are dismissed. In the past, doctors simply did not think it was their role to extend the limits of the medical profession, and most accepted, as an adequate reward, the instant and enormous gratification that comes in healing the wounds of war without demanding any further involvement, without, in most circumstances, even staying long enough to critically assess their own efforts.

For example, health workers have long embraced the comforting concept of medical neutrality without carefully weighing its political implications. In World War II, few seemed to seriously question whether the Red Cross was morally right to adhere to their treasured code of political neutrality by distributing biscuits and food parcels in Auschwitz or Buchenwald while never criticizing or publicly condemning Nazi methods. Do today's humanitarian workers have the courage to question whether the very aid they deliver is being used to foster oppression or as a tool for ethnic cleansing? Do they merely prolong the agonies of war when they innocently contribute supplies without being aware that their help may perpetuate the power of evil leaders, as happened in the Goma refugee camps after the Rwanda genocide? Is it ever possible to stay professionally aloof from such practical political, and deeply moral, questions, especially ones that are so predictable?

Humanitarian assistance in international conflicts always has a political dimension. This should not be a source for embarrassment – it is a simple fact of life. Politics affects everyone in the chain – from the donors, to the distributors, to the recipients. One has only to look at the funding of the large voluntary agencies in the United States to appreciate the political dimension. CARE, for example, seen as the compassionate voluntary effort of concerned American individuals, receives the vast amount of its budget from USAID and other government sources, and the person who pays the piper can surely call the tune. Who gets food, and when, and for how long, is based on political factors.

America's multimillion dollar effort to assist oppressed Kurds in Northern Iraq – codenamed *Operation Provide Comfort* – was canceled within a week when our favored Kurdish faction decided they were safer with local Iraqi rather than Iranian protection. The cover of humanitarian concern was blown away by the cold winds of political reality. I was in Somalia when President Bush sent in 28,000 troops to help the starving masses. TV cameras and reporters were flown to Mogadishu, in advance, so they could record the troop landings for the evening television news/entertainment. One year, and $4 billion later, we left a country in chaos.

One can seriously argue what good, if any, came from this whole sad experience. Anarchy still reigns in Somalia, but the attention of a fickle world, overwhelmed by other tragedies, has moved on. Somalia is no longer newsworthy. Political judgements dictated our arrival and departure schedules. The knowledge or insights of academics and health workers who knew the people and the customs of the Somalis seemed to matter very little to those who defined our "national interest." The United States had entered Somalia because of a putative concern about the health of a starving populace. The foreign policy results of a noble gesture gone awry were far more profound than the scenes of famine we were supposed to eliminate. As with Vietnam, a great tragedy flowed from America's failed involvement in Somalia. Its relationship with the United Nations unraveled with catastrophic implications for future international humanitarian missions.

When civil unrest in Rwanda erupted in 1994, the Secretary-General of the UN literally begged the Security Council to send a peacekeeping force. The United States led the opposition to this appeal because it did not wish to cross what was now called the "Mogadishu line," the commitment of American forces under a UN flag in a foreign country. Within the next two months, 800,000 Rwandans were hacked to death with machetes, and the churches and lakes were clogged with the corpses of innocent victims of neglect. The world knew what was happening and we watched but did little except debate procedures, arguing over the methods of payment that must be assured for surplus transport, before we would become involved.

Fifty years after the Holocaust, after the United States joined in the chorus of "never again," it silently observed the most intense months of genocide in the history of mankind. Then, the most massive movement of refugees ever recorded began; in a single day over a million people poured into the small town of Goma in DRC. Very late in the course of the disaster, the same donor governments that had refused to help months before, now poured $2 billion into an uncoordinated relief effort that resulted in sustaining the very murderers we had failed to stop when the genocide began.

The Somali and Rwanda experiences were disastrous, and my own articles on health and foreign policy reflect those debacles. Working with land mine victims amidst the desolation of Somalia in the early 1990s, I was convinced one could not merely write another book or research paper. It was time to develop a new approach, demand changes, embarrass, if necessary, political leaders until they responded appropriately to the realities of conflicts and disasters as seen on the ground, in the midst of conflict, by those who had unique access to the people involved. It was time to be more assertive – for the sake of my country as well as for the Somali amputees I had come to know so well.

At the same time, former US Secretary of State Cyrus Vance accepted my invitation to deliver one of the Distinguished International Health Lectures to this College. In a reflective answer to a student's question, he noted, with self-amazement, that this had been the first time he had ever mentioned health in a speech. His whole background and approach were rooted in a Cold War ethos where military alliances, power blocks and geopolitical factors determined whom, and to what carefully measured degree, his nation helped overseas. But he now observed that, in the post Cold War era, it was the differences between the North and the South, between the haves and the have nots, that most frequently precipitated regional and world conflicts. The health worker could no longer be a peripheral partner in diplomacy.

Shortly thereafter a small group of diplomats and physicians decided to form a voluntary organization – The Center for International Humanitarian Cooperation (CIHC) in order to promote the role of health in diplomacy. I edited *Preventive Diplomacy: Stopping Wars Before They Start*, in which leading politicians and statesmen from around the world joined with humanitarian workers in applying the methods and approaches of public health, as well as the metaphors of medicine, to the ancient but soft art of diplomacy. If preventive diplomacy is to replace traditional reactive diplomacy, there must be a fundamental change in our national mind set. At present only problems that attain crisis proportion seem to attract the attention of politicians or diplomats.

Our leaders simply are not attuned to deal with incipient disorder at a time when prevention is possible. Public figures are obsessed with dramatic solutions, with a fire brigade approach that assures a continuation of catastrophes. In preventive medicine one begins by searching for fundamental causes, for the etiology of a disease, and for techniques that can interrupt transmission before serious signs and symptoms become obvious and irreversible damage occurs. One should be able to adapt this approach to the epidemiology of warfare. The origins of conflict clearly lie in incubating prejudices and injustices that inevitably breed hatred and violence. But how rarely are these evil forces exposed early enough, or fought with effective tools, before predictable disaster strikes? If a fatal disease threatens to spread, health experts devise control programs based on careful research and laboratory experiments, sophisticated statistical studies and models, field trials and double blind surveys, that try to minimize biases and biologic variants which so often contaminate the best intentioned projects. When deaths do occur, scrupulous postmortem analyses are customary so that the faults and failures of the past become the building blocks for a better approach to the future.

Diplomatic exercises should be subjected to similar probes and autopsies. Nations, particularly great powers and international organizations, must become humble enough to learn from failed efforts rather than merely defending their actions and hiding their errors. If there are new actors in world conflicts, and a new global environment created by, among other factors, a communications revolution, then the therapeutics of international diplomacy must also change. Such views are expounded in *Preventive Diplomacy*, by widely respected diplomats and humanitarian workers whose idealism and passion for peace are grounded in the very real world of wars and disasters.

The very goal of creating a new diplomacy, of thinking that one can stop wars before they start, may seem like innocent dreams to sceptics. But one has only to consider the changing nature, and number, of global conflicts to appreciate the importance of this initiative. In World War I over 90% of the casualties were soldiers; today over 90% of the victims in most current wars are innocent civilians caught in a web of ancient hatreds, with whole populations struggling to survive in a world where a decline in the security of national sovereignty, and a collapse of the rules of civil society, is matched by a rise in ethnicity, by the incredible cruelty of civil wars, by man-made famine, by the widespread use of rape as a weapon of war, by land mines that scar the earth long after battles are fought, by the forced displacement of tens of millions who wander without hope in 'failed states' that no longer exist, by a generation who have come to accept as normal so much needless violence, brutality and suffering.

It is time, for both pragmatic and symbolic reasons, to recognize health and humanitarian issues as central to foreign policy. In diplomacy as in public health, we must build a system that guards against known dangers, and tries to more effectively contain the inevitable threats to peace. We must find alternatives to the confrontational practices that still characterize most relations between states. There is now a chance that the principle of prevention may take its place as a significant improvement over inaction or coercion in dealing with conflicts.

By emphasizing the basic health and humanitarian concerns of preventive diplomacy, the United Nations could capitalize on its unique role, as the sole acceptable vehicle for all peoples and States, to improve essential early warning systems, to develop more effective regional organizations, and to fully involve both governmental and non-governmental agencies in a new form of diplomacy that is not predicated simply on power politics or military might. Even after conflicts have begun, this new diplomacy, based on a philosophy that focuses on root causes and promotes early involvement, can help de-escalate violence and hasten the restoration of peace. The use of medical metaphors to define and describe the goals–as well as the complexities–of foreign policy might also make sense to a cynical and confused citizenry.

Almost 500 years ago, in a small book that remains a classic text on politics and diplomacy, Machiavelli shrewdly employed the semantics of health to explain a fundamental tenet of governing; he wrote:

'*When trouble is sensed well in advance, it can easily be remedied; if you wait for it to show it, any medicine will be too late because the disease will have become incurable. As the doctors say of a wasting disease, to start with it is easy to cure but difficult to diagnose; after a time, unless it has been diagnosed and treated at the outset, it becomes easy to diagnose but difficult to cure. So it is in politics.'*

The United Nations, however imperfect or structurally handicapped, represents a fundamental, if tentative, step toward a world society and away from the anarchy of unaccountable sovereign nations. For the United Nations preventive diplomacy is an absolute imperative. It provides an approach that could allow the UN to regain the moral base that was the dream of its Founders, to be an organization that would help prevent war by coordinating the efforts of the entire family of nations. In the current climate of global adhocracy the UN inherits the most intractable problems, and then is blamed for failing to solve conflicts often caused, ignored or abandoned by the big power observers. The ever-escalating cost of UN military interventions distorts the primary mission and drains the resources and morale of an organization founded to beat swords into ploughshares, to help create a healthy and peaceful world.

Today's political climate, for some similar and some different reasons, provides another opportunity to alter the way the developed nations are perceived in many parts of the world, especially in turbulent, poor nations where internal conflict is almost constant. Political, military and humanitarian interests are not mutually exclusive; in fact, they form the triad on which international intervention must be built. France, stimulated by the work of Médecins Sans Frontières (MSF) has already appointed a formal Minister of Humanitarian Affairs. It is time the United States fully recognizes the critical benefits and creative balance that humanitarian actions offer, so that they become an official and proud, not peripheral, part of our foreign policy.

There are no final answers; there cannot be in our finite and imperfect state. In public health all the old challenges remain, and new diseases seem to constantly emerge. The explosion of drug resistant tuberculosis is a classic result of public complacency to an old but resurgent infectious plague; new viruses and environmental changes continue to challenge our capacity to adapt and respond. So too, in the endless search for world peace, we should not be surprised that our noble goal proves elusive. But simply to accept failure, to impotently adhere to an outmoded approach that denies the unique wonder of the Western world would be a tragedy both for our own nations and for those around the world who look to us for a new direction in a new century.

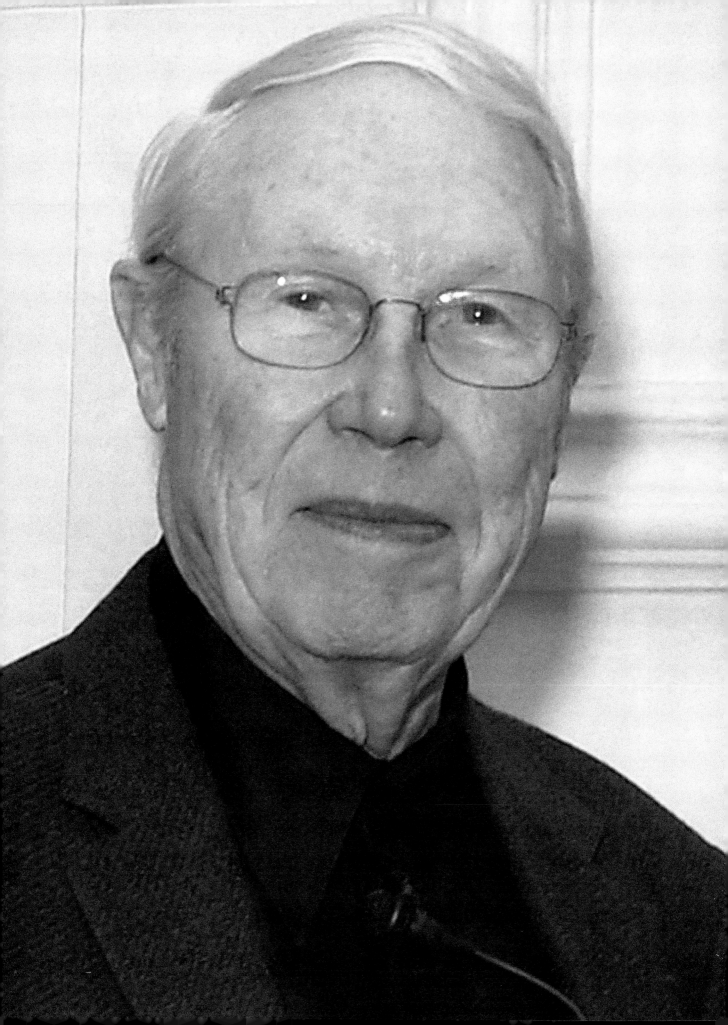

Louis Le Brocquy

His Distinguished International Lecture was delivered in the College on November 14, 2005.

Over 30 years ago, in the Introduction to the Catalog for Louis Le Brocquy's first major show in the United States, I noted the relationship of his art to medicine: "As a young man in Dublin he worked for a time as an illustrator for a neurosurgeon, attending operations and trying to record the appearance of diseased pituitary glands in the hidden recesses of the brain. From this 'terrible experience' he became fascinated by the mind of man and noted, *…here I am myself, forty years later, still trying in my own way to enter behind the face, the skull, the os frontis, to discover another interior landscape.*" He is universally acknowledged as one of the greatest Irish artists, and I am proud to have called him a friend. He died at the age of 95 in 2012.

The Human Head: Notes on Painting and Awareness
Louis Le Brocquy

When I first jotted down these thoughts in 1979 I was preoccupied by Celtic image of the human head as a magic box containing consciousness. Today, I find myself still groping beyond human appearance towards the impalpable reality that lies within us.

As a painter, I have always been concerned with the one or other aspect of the body as an image of the human being. In recent years I have turned more specifically to the poet's head as an image of human consciousness.

The human body is a constantly recurring theme of both the poet and painter, but their two arts—each a whole continent of consciousness—do not touch directly, I think, at any point. They have no common frontier, no bridge other than their shared state of aesthetic *awareness*. Turning, then, in the direction of that bridge, I shall try—as a painter—to speak of painting and awareness.

William Blake believed that "man's perceptions are not bounded by organs of perception." Evidently painting lies within these bounds. Yet I think of the art of painting as another way of seeing, another approach to reality—another porthole, as it were, in the submerged bathysphere of our consciousness.

In the context of our everyday lives, painting must be regarded as an entirely different form of awareness, for an essential quality of art is its alienation, its *otherness*. In art at its most profound level, actuality—exterior reality—is seen to be relevant, parallel, but remote or curiously dislocated.

Where actuality plays an immediate role as in photographic images, in kite flying, in Christo's "Running Fence" or other forms of recording, descriptive or environmental arts, aesthetic perception and elation may be experienced but scarcely, I think, deep recurrent insight. Such insight, when it occurs in painting, is due, I suggest, to an essential ambivalence in the role of the paint itself, which is characteristic of significant painting. It may be relevant here to quote from something I wrote in London in 1956:

Since painting first interested me, I have been drawn to a constant tradition which I think of as central to this old European art. This implies a peculiar use of oil paint; not to symbolize, not to describe the object, nor to realize an abstract image but rather to allow the paint, while insisting upon its own palpable nature, to reconstitute the object of one's experience: to metamorphose into the image of an apple, a sky, a human back.

This is an indefinable, a mysterious process and is accordingly rare. Giorgione, Titian, Tintoretto used paint in this way. Caravaggio sent it on its way to Spain to Velázquez. Rembrandt epitomized it. Turner pushed it to its metaphysical limits. Watteau, Chardin, Delacroix, Courbet, Manet, Monet and Cézanne were among its great French exponents.

In certain works of all these, the paint (with its qualities of color, tone and texture) has been transformed into the experienced object.

Obversely, the image of the object has become paint. This dichotomy, this tension pulls taut the nerves of insight. Reality is stripped down to a deeper layer and the ordinary is seen to be marvellous.

Indeed you may say that such a paint-image is itself a manifestation of the mind-beyond-reason, grasping at the natural fact which it mirrors. I think of Ahab's cry in Moby Dick:

O Nature and O Soul of Man! How far beyond all utterances are your linked analogies! Not the smallest atom stirs or lives on matter, but has its cunning duplicate in mind.

And then again I ask myself whether this "cunning duplicate in mind" may not be another way of naming the *claritas* of Thomas Aquinas's definition of beauty, which—as Mark Patrick Hederman has pointed out—James Joyce translates as *radiance*. Joyce writes in *Portrait of a Young Man*:

The aesthetic image is first luminously apprehended as self bounded and self-contained upon the immeasurable background of space and time which it is not… The connotation of the word "claritas" is rather vague. Aquinas uses a term which seems to be inexact. It baffled me for a long time. It would lead you to believe that he had in mind symbolism or idealism, the supreme quality of human beauty being a light from some other world… But when you have apprehended that basket as one thing and have then analyzed it as a thing, you make the only synthesis which logically and esthetically permissible. You see that it is that thing and no other. The radiance of which he speaks is the scholastic quidditas, the whatness of a thing.

Here Joyce is presumably thinking specifically in terms of writing, of poetry. But it is evident that this "whatness" of the image is the equally the essence of the art of painting.

For, contrary to a generally held view, I think that painting is not in any direct sense a means of communication or self-expression. For me at any rate, it is groping towards an image, a "whatness."

When you are painting you are trying to discover, to uncover, to reveal. I sometimes think of the activity of painting as a kind of archaeology – an archaeology of the spirit. As in archaeology, accident continually plays an important part. The painter, like the archaeologist, is a *watcher,* a supervisor of accident; patiently disturbing the surface of things until a significant accident becomes apparent, recognizing it, conserving this as best he can while provoking the possibility of further accident. In this way a whole image, a *whatness*, may with luck gradually emerge almost spontaneously.

Thus, what counts in painting is, I believe, recognition of significant accident within a larger preoccupation and *not* dexterity and skill and calculated imposition. Ironically enough I myself have frequently been reproached with possessing too much dexterity, too much technical skill. Recently I was given a rather dramatic opportunity to disprove this charge when, after a bone-grafting operation to my right hand, my whole arm was immobilized in plaster for a number of months. During this period the images which emerged under my ignorant left hand were in fact in no way distinguishable from those induced by my practical right hand. Neither better nor worse.

Some seventeen years ago I was still painting the torso as an image of the human presence, when I stumbled into what I call a blind year – a year in which I had no luck, in which no image emerged. At the end of that year I destroyed forty-three bad paintings. As you can imagine, I was by then in a bad way myself, when my wife Anne Madden – herself a painter – brought me to Paris as to a place of discovery. And there indeed I did discover at the Musée de l'Homme, the Polynesian image of the human head, which like the Celtic image which I discovered the following year, represented for me—as perhaps for these two widely different cultures—the mysterious box which contains the spirit: the outer reality of the invisible interior world of consciousness.

In Dublin, over sixty years ago today, the great physicist, Erwin Schroedinger, astonished me with the thought:

Consciousness is a singular of which the plural is unknown and what appears to be plurality is merely a series of different aspects of this one thing.

Much later in Provence, faced with the Celto-Ligurian head cult of Entremont and Roquepertuse, I asked myself if it were not perhaps this "singular" which so preoccupied our barbarian ancestors.

Such a concept of an autonomous, disseminated consciousness surpassing individual personality would, I imagine, tend to produce an ambiguity involving a dislocation of our individual conception of time (within which coming and going, beginning and end, are normally regarded) and confronting this "normal" view with an alternative, contrary sense of simultaneity or timelessness; switching the linear conception of time to which we are accustomed to a circular concept returning upon itself, as in *Finnegans Wake*.

Likewise, if indeed the aesthetic image in a painting by Rembrandt is illuminated by Joyce's *radiance* or *whatness*, and if that revelation *whatness* is achieved by an ambivalence in the role of the paint (involving a transmogrification of the paint itself in to the image and vice versa), then these circumstances also may be said to produce that timeless or para-temporal quality, which we instinctively recognize in a painting by Rembrandt.

It would therefore seem that the realization of the aesthetic image or *whatness* of things, outside and to one side of the linear progress of time, is an essential characteristic of the art of painting and, I imagine, of art generally.

In the modern world, however, we appear to resist such significant *integrating* imagery, which was more evident perhaps in past cultures, wherein people seem to have regarded the passage of time rather more ambivalently, as being at once relative to their personal predicament and to a larger cosmology.

It would appear that this ambivalent attitude to time was especially linked to the ancient Celtic or Gallic world, and there is further evidence that it persists to some extent in the Celtic mind today. It is consistent, I think, with Yeat's *tragic* view of life—an essentially cosmologic and aristocratic attitude in opposition to the narrow expediency of the "greasy till":

We Irish, born into the ancient sect
But thrown upon this filthy modern tide
And by its formless spawning fury wrecked
Climb to our proper dark, that we may trace
The lineaments of a plummet-measured face.

In my own small world of painting I myself have learned from the canvas that emergence and disappearance—twin phenomena of time—are ambivalent, that one implies the other and that the state or matrix within which they co-exist dissolves the normal sense of time, producing a characteristic *stillness*, inherent in the art of painting.

After a number of years I recall Beckett's Watt, regarding from a gate the distant figure of a man or a woman (or could it be a priest or a nun?) which appeared to be advancing by slow degrees from the horizon, only surprisingly "without any interruption of its motions" to disappear over it instead. Here going is confounded—if not identified—with coming, backwards with forwards. The film returns the diver to the diving board. The procession of present events is reversed, stilled.

Elsewhere in *Finnegans Wake* does not the fallen Finnegan become "Finn Macool lying beside the Liffey, his head at Howth, his feet a Phoenix Park, his wife beside him, *watching the microcosmic 'fluid succession of presents' go by like a river of life?*"

And is not Yeat's circular lunar system of re-incarnation—mimicked by the winding stair of Thoor Ballylee, climbed and descended repeatedly—itself a formal arrangement of this *fluid succession of presents*, which "the past assuredly implies," of time-consciousness in this profoundly Celtic sense? Is this indeed the underlying ambivalence which we in Ireland tend to stress; the continued presence of the historic past, the indivisibility of birth and funeral, spanning the apparent chasm between past and present, between consciousness and fact?

Not long ago I had the good fortune to decorate with ink paintings—shadows thrown by the text—Thomas Kinsella's marvelous translation, from 8th and 12th century Irish MSS, of the central Irish legendary epic, Táin Bó Cualigne. On its cover is a simple brush drawing, a minor image of the virtual shield of the fabulous hero, Cúchulainn, and indeed of this archetypal Celtic warrior himself who, Christ-like, chose an early explosive death that we might receive the unending fallout of his substance. But paradoxically this explosive, emergent image can equally be interpreted as implosive, accretive. Thus conversely it can become the mythical Crane Bag of the Irish sea-god Mannanán Mac Lir, a magic sack made from the skin of a woman who had been transformed into a heron or crane: a legendary receptacle sunk in the sea, gathering or expelling its treasures with the tides, breathing and exhaling like a lung "a fluid succession of presents," day-conscious/night-conscious, like Ulysses and Finnegan, or like a living human head, image of the while in the part, the old synecdochism of the Celt.

But turn to the heads themselves in the powerful, shattered sculpture of the Celto-Ligurian Entremont, or to the later multiple heads within the "plummet-measure" face of Romanesque Confert in County Galway. At once person and stone bosses, both durable and timeless, forever emerging and receding, they signify a profound paradox, a balanced ambivalence, a succession of present moments dredged up from time, spread out before us without beginning or end.

For over fifteen years I have tried to draw from the depths of paper, or from the white canvas, a human face. As I have remarked, this quiet activity has little to do with communication, or with self-expression for that matter. It aims rather to make visible a lurking image, to identify, to name some trace or aspect of a personal reality. Which means to me the giving of a *possible* form to that which is impalpable or interiorized. For I imagine that reality is that which is possible, conceivable and not merely what is actual, phenomenal.

So when painting, I try not to impose myself. Discoveries are made – such as they are – while painting. The painting itself dictates and, although the resultant image may seem rhetorical to some it appears to me to be almost autonomous, having emerged under one's hands and not because of them. A subjectively conceived image, deliberately imposed by the painter, may ne represented easily enough. A conventional, popular image of W.B. Yeats is immediately recognizable to those who share it. Such a conceived image may be sought and repeatedly rediscovered in the flux and movement of life, but what of a photograph where factual appearance is momentarily and permanently stilled and which sometimes defies identification with the known conceptual image? If two contemporary photographs of Yeats provide acceptable images of him, a third does not. For the successive factual appearances of each one of us are necessarily dissimilar, since each one of us has many layers, many aspects, and none more than Yeats. In the 100 studies towards an image of W.B. Yeats, which were exhibited in 1976 at the Musée d'Art Moderne de la Ville de Paris, I therefore tried as uncritically as I could to allow different aspects of Yeat's head to emerge. These I recalled largely from photographs taken throughout his lifetime and, for the most part, without referring to them directly. Where I have worked from them directly, I have consulted two or more at the same time and—since these photographs bear little consistent resemblance to each other—I have encouraged differing and sometimes contradictory images to emerge spontaneously in order, as it were, to exorcise my own rather conventional memory of Yeats and in the hope of discovering a more immediate image—stilled and free of circumstance—underlying the ever-changing aspect of this phenomenal Irishman.

My mother was a friend of the Yeats family in Dublin and so when I was a boy, I was fairly familiar with "W.B.'s" appearance and with his extremely impressive manner.

In 1938 I left Ireland and my grandfather's business to become a painter. Having no training, I studied at museums in London, Paris, Venice and Geneva, where the great Prado collection was then exhibited, having been sent from Madrid by the elected government, in face of Franco's artillery.

The following year, when Yeats died in Roquebrune, I was painting a few kilometers away in a minute house on the Cap Martin. To my lasting regret I knew neither of his presence nor of his death. I am conscious that the long series of studies towards an image of Yeats, which I made thirty-five years later, was in some sense a personal adventure to try to rediscover, to touch the fringes of his enormous personality; to enter perhaps into the interior landscape which lay behind "those ancient glittering eyes."

For me, as perhaps for our Celtic and Gallic ancestors, the human head can be regarded ambivalently as a box which hold the spirit prisoner, but which may also free it transparently within the face. Paradoxically, as we know, the face is at once a mask which hides the spirit and a revelation of this spirit.

As I conceive it, there lies behind the face an interior landscape which the painter tries to discover. But I know too that this landscape may also be a reflection from within the painter himself. In this sense you peer at this Other, searching for a larger image of yourself, just as Yeats, the contemplative man, peered at his own antithetic mask, his opposite – the *swift indifferent* man – and tried to bring that opposite to the surface of his personality.

Yeats was, I imagine, an essentially interiorized mind witnessing the slow dissolution of an outward-looking era.

As we know, since the renaissance and until the beginning of the last century our imagery has remained largely outward-looking and evidently equated with exterior phenomena.

Prior to the Renaissance, however, it was though that reality was to be found within the mind itself, within those conceptual images of a world transformed by religious belief.

In our own time, true enough, our popular imaging is largely based on the objective photograph. Nevertheless, since the beginning of the 20th century, a profound change occurred in painting when, inspired by Cézanne, Picasso, Matisse and other visionary artists, we awoke to the renewed conceptual vision of our age.

Likewise in literature, Beckett, while still in his twenties, expressed "…awareness of the new thing that has happened, namely the breakdown of the object… (the) rupture of the lines of communication…" and "…the space which intervenes between (the artist) and the world of objects…".

Today we begin to understand anew the nature of this ambiguous space. To see is to transform. Art is a transformer. The hand can act as an independent being to bring about the emergence of the image. The painter must wait for this without imposing his ideas, watching intensely and critically for what may happen. I am convinced that Paleolithic man acted in this way. He was an artist, but above all a seer. There is a brain in the hand. The hand in the cave of Pech-Merle is a personality. A hand-print is a personality. A footprint is only a trace, an imprint. Why?

When I am working I do not think, other than in a narrow technical sort of way. Painting is a form of thought within which a wider intelligence plays no important part. It has its own logic. For me, at any rate, there is no question of invention. In painting you can only hope for discovery. Invention for me is *recognition*. When you are painting, marks combine to form *objets trouvés* which may be recognized. You try to preserve these and to induce something further. If that works, an entire image may emerge. If not, it will fail.

When I was painting Yeats he was my Virgil, my guide in this Other-world. His image gave me stability, reference. However I stayed, trying to realize that image – to make it palpable – he held me on his trial. At times I even had the feeling of touching him. At times I was the charlatan who toyed with the apparition of Yeats, as one might conjure up the dead in spiritualism.

You may well object that such an approach is merely subjective. But then the art of the painter depends upon an essentially subjective process. It is even true that the painter continually tends to paint his self-portrait in all things, since what he tries objectively to draw up from the depth of his canvas lies really somewhere in his own head.

For, such intimate knowledge as you may try to attain of another human being through his works, all that you can know of him, passes behind the billowing curtain of his face. And if this curtain be carefully drawn aside, you are liable sometimes to find only poor traces of yourself.

Nonetheless I believe that the hand can lead us away from ourselves and discover our *mask*; that which is other to ourselves, outside or superior to ourselves. I imagine that Rembrandt displayed the highest intelligence in projecting objectively perceived ideas of himself into his self-portraits. In this sense they are not strictly self-portraits at all, but rather portraits of a man he saw in his mirror, the enlisted sufferer whose endurance he well knew. Perhaps this is the reason for the poignant humility of these works.

During the last five years I have painted in various media three long series of studies—of Yeats, of James Joyce and of Federico Garcia Lorca. Although I knew Yeats personally, as a boy might know an uncle or school-master, I have best learned to know each one of these great artists through their work, through my own glimpse of the envisaged worlds which lie behind their three exceptional foreheads.

In the case of Lorca, I have been moved to add to the series of paintings several further studies in bronze of his forehead, *Os frontis*, in an attempt to touch that broad tabernacle of his vision.

Oh, city of gypsies!...
Who could see you and forget?
Let them seek you on my brow
The play of moon and sand.

I am aware that that vision lies far away from my own familiar country which gave birth to Yeats and Joyce. Federico, far away, lending his Iberian temperament and his voice to the unheard cries of his people, echoing with what he called his "astonished flesh."

For me an Irishman, it was curiously enough the plays of Synge that provided the key to an understanding of Lorca's fierce, lyrical world.

It was only recently that I was told by Mark Mortimer in Paris that Lorca knew and admired the works of John Millington Synge.

Ever since I rediscovered for myself the image of the head, I have painted studies of James Joyce. I have never known Joyce, but am bound to him as a Dubliner. For it is said that no-one from that city can quite escape its microcosmic world, and I am certainly no exception. Joyce is the apotheosis, the archetype of our kind and it seems to me that in him – behind the volatile arrangement of his features – lies his unique evocation of that small city, large as life and therefore poignant everywhere. But to me, a Dublin man peering at Joyce, a particular nostalgia is added to the universal "epiphany" and this perhaps enables me to grope for something of my own experience within the everchanging landscape of his face, within the various and contradictory photographs of his head, within my bronze death-mask of him and, I suppose, within the recesses of my own mind.

Thus almost 10 studies towards an image of James Joyce have emerged in one medium or another. It remains an unending task. For to attempt today a portrait, a single static image of a great artist like Joyce seems to me futile as well as impertinent. Long conditioned by photography, the cinema and psychology, we now perceive the human individual as facetted, kinetic.

And so I have tried as objectively as possible to draw, from the depths of paper or canvas, changing and even contradictory traces of James Joyce; images jerked into coherence by a series of scrutinized accidents, impelled by my curiosity to discover something of the man and, within him, the inverted mirror-room of my own Dublin experience.

I myself therefore see these studies rather as an indefinite series without beginning or end and thus perhaps in tendency counter-Renaissance, as in a sense was also Joyce himself. Possibly their multiple identity may represent a more medieval or even Celtic viewpoint, cyclic rather than linear, repetitive yet simultaneous and, above all, inconclusive.

They have been for me an adventure—an adventure of discovery—and not without its perils and its fears. We are told that the great *naïf* painter, Douanier Rousseau, stood terror-struck outside the door of his studio, summoning up his courage to re-enter and confront the marvelous lion which broods over his sleeping gypsy.

I confess I felt something of the same fearful hesitation on returning to the door of my own studio in France and to the multiple photographic and other images of Joyce which filled it. I am unable to account for this sudden aversion which overcame me, other than as a fear perhaps of re-entering into certain painful aspects of his temperament, of his unending difficulties. In painting Yeats, or Lorca, I never experienced this recoil, this passing shudder.

But once back in the studio and facing again those images of James Joyce my fear gave way to those larger feelings of reverence, compassion and wonder which we all share in face of that unique boat-shaped head—the raised poop of the forehead, the jutting bow of the jaw—within which he made his heroic voyage, his *navigatio.*

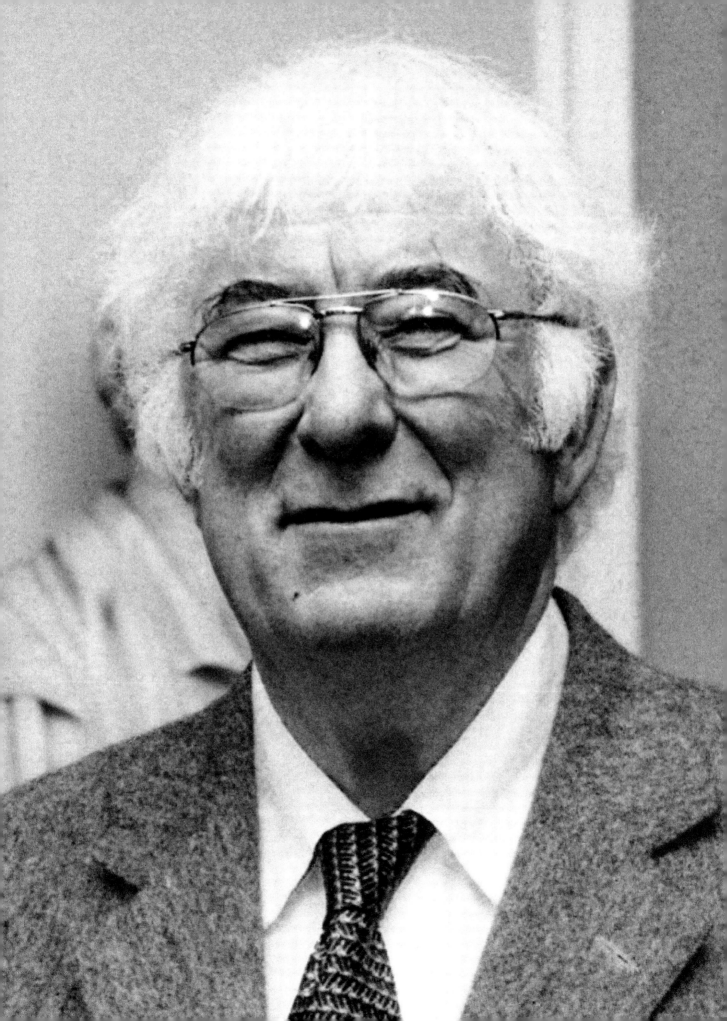

Seamus Heaney

His Distinguished International Lecture was delivered in the College on November 5, 2001.

Seamus Heaney won the Nobel Prize for Literature in 1995. Born in County Derry, Northern Ireland, his poetry drew universal lessons from rural Irish experiences. He first published poems in 1962, and by the end of a long, very distinguished, career he had 13 volumes of poetry, and numerous other books of plays, translations, and essays. He was Professor and Poet in Residence for many years at both Harvard and Oxford Universities. He was the best known poet of his generation, and his books accounted for a staggering percentage of all poetry books sold. When Seamus died in 2013, the President of Ireland, Michael D. Higgins, captured my own feelings of loss – "What those of us who had the privilege of his friendship and presence will miss is the extraordinary depth and warmth of his personality."

The Whole Thing:
On the Good of Poetry
Seamus Heaney

Previous speakers in this series have been people whose contributions to the good of the world have been crucial, practical and admirable: peacemakers, healers, researchers into new ways of combating disease, campaigners against the old evils of war and pestilence. All these lecturers were active workers in the field of what is now called "international health," and they came here to speak at the invitation of Professor Kevin Cahill, the man who has been most influential in the development of this concept of international health, and most important not only in giving it theoretical definition, but also in helping to secure its practical implementation as part of the effort towards a braver, newer world.

It seemed right, therefore, that my own lecture should be about the part poetry can be said to play in such an effort and such an evolution. Hence its subtitle, "the good of poetry," a phrase which on its own can sound out of place linguistically. I mean to say that in English we are more used to hearing the words "the good of..." in contexts that are interrogative rather than affirmative. Usually we are asking *"What's* the good of?" this or that—of crying over spilt milk or shutting the stable door when the horse is gone, of attending conferences against racism or of writing poetry. For once, however, I want to be affirmative, maybe even a bit demonstrative, since I am going to begin by reading a poem of my own.

This was written over thirty years ago, after I had heard a piece of music played at the Queen's University Festival in 1968. On that occasion, the Irish composer Sean O'Riada was the

Festival's special guest, and there was a special thrill about the way he brought traditional musicians into the art music context, the way *bainin* jackets displaced bow ties and a spirit of carnival threatened to disrupt the composure and conventions of the concert hall. One of the tunes his group played was an arrangement of a haunting slow air called in Irish "port na bpúcai." Which could be translated as "the music of the spirits," and my poem basically retells the story O'Riada told by way of introduction to the performance. According to the folklore, the tune was first heard by a fiddler on one of Blasket Islands, coming in on the night wind over the sound of the waves:

The Given Note

On the most westerly Blasket
In a dry stone hut
He got this air out of the night.

Strange noises were heard
By others who followed, bits of a tune
Coming in on loud weather

Though nothing like melody.
He blamed their fingers and ears
As unpractised, their fiddling easy

For he had gone into the island

And brought back the whole thing.
The house throbbed like his full violin.

So whether he calls it spirit music or not,
I don't care. He took it
Out of wind off mid-Atlantic.

Still he maintains, from nowhere.
It comes off the bow gravely,
Rephrases itself into the air.

The story at the centre of this is an old one, reappearing in many versions and many contexts. It has an archetypal appeal. It prompts us to remember the voice speaking from the whirlwind. Or the mighty wind heard by the apostles when tongues of flame descended on them in the upper room and they emerged from the place like men drunk on new wine, speaking in tongues. It prompts us to reflect on music's relationship to the ineffable, and by analogy, on poetry's link to the transcendent. It reminds us that the spirit itself is synonymous with breath, that the word inspiration has behind it the idea of air being breathed or blown in. It calls up Shelley's great "Ode to the West Wind," where the poet cries out, "Be thou, Spirit fierce, / My spirit! Be thou me, impetuous one!" and William Wordsworth's invocation of the blowing breeze as a sort of angelic messenger (at the start of his autobiographical *magnum opus, The Prelude*). Behind the simplicity of the country fiddler's tale, in other words, there lie the grandeur and resonance of biblical narrative, of classical etymology and philosophy, and the more recent poetics of the Romantic movement.

So much for storm and inspiration. Now, however, I want to pay attention to that phrase "the whole thing," which I chose deliberately as the title of the lecture, but which I used without any conscious deliberation when I was writing "The Given Note" in Belfast in 1968. I used it in the poem intuitively because it sounded right, because it fell like a plumb line in the ear, because its rhythmic and phonetic weight dropped safely and, in all senses, soundly, into place. "He blamed their fingers and ear /As unpractised, their fiddling easy / For he had gone alone into the island /And brought back the whole thing": it still seems to me that the meaning and the cadence come to rest there, settle and steady themselves surely in the verbal order of things—and you will understand that in saying so I don't mean to take any personal credit to myself for this particular arrangement of the lines. You can hear with your own ears that the language itself was disposed to come out and come down in exactly those terms, as if in obedience to some pulse or wave pattern at work not only in my ear but in the general ear, in the very life-lines of spoken English. And I would argue that at a primal level, the good of poetry resides in just such a sensation of rightness, a sensation you might characterize by saying, "It did me good just to hear it."

But the words of a language are bound to keep faith not only with sound but with sense; as well as being keyed to certain instinctive registers. They are answerable to meaning. And it was the meaning stored up in the phrase "the whole thing" that made me pay attention when I thought of it as a title for this lecture.

In the old thirteen-volume *Oxford English Dictionary,* three complete folio-sized pages—altogether nine columns of definition and citation—are devoted to the word "whole," but these are preceded by a list of etymological cognates which I'll list briefly here (and probably mispronounce). First comes the main root-word, the Anglo-Saxon *hal,* with its immediate relations, Old Swedish and Old Frisian *hel,* the variously spelled Old Dutch and Old High German and Old Norse cognates *heil/heel* or *geheel*, all of these being traced back to an Indo-European root—*quoilos,* and then in turn—*quoilos* is seen to branch out into related terms in Old Slavic. Old Irish *cel* also makes an appearance, a word meaning omen, related in its way to the Old Norse *heil*, which when feminine meant happiness or good luck. What holds all these variants together, of course, is the general meaning of being in good condition, sound, free from damage, intact, total, unimpaired. Then, proceeding from those root meanings, from all the various sounds and senses of *whole*—we arrive at the cluster of words and meanings in *hale* and *health* and *heal,* and these in turn bring us back from the columns of the dictionary to the healing grounds of the College of Surgeons and this afternoon's lecture in the International Health Series.

The virtue of poetry, of art in general, resides in the fact that it is first and foremost a whole thing, a thing formally and feelingly sound, right within itself, a thing to which the ultimate response—if not always the immediate response—is "yes". And this yes comes from an assent that is as bodily as it is anything else. The viewer, the listener, the audience recognizes that something has come through to them intact, or perhaps better say they recognize that something has been *brought* through to them and brought home. In fact, one of the ways you might distinguish between the categories of natural and artistic beauty would be to say that the natural *comes* home to you but the artistic is *brought* home. And as I have often said before, this bringing home, this moving of a certain force through a certain distance, constitutes the work of art.

To speak of the work of art is to speak of one of two things, either the action which brings the work into being or the finished job, be it a poem or a picture or a fugue. What I want to stress here is the importance of the first of these things, namely the technical aspect, the doing of the job, the actual business of carrying through a process of composition. I want to emphasize the fact that the discovery of wholeness is not a mystical matter; it is instead the result of a worker's specialized skills and heightened intuitions being brought to bear deliberately and intently; or to put it another way, a poet's intelligence and cognitive faculties are never more alive than during those moments when he appears to be off in a world of his own, absorbed in the creative trance, preoccupied with the dream-work. And surgeons, I am sure, will see parallels here between that kind of absorption and the kind of concentration required from them as they practise their own intensely preoccupied art.

In this regard, indeed, I am always reminded of a story I heard from the late Sean Ronan, a distinguished servant of the Department of Foreign Affairs whom I first met when he was Ireland's ambassador in Japan. Anyway, Sean was a wise and funny man and one of the instructive tales he told had to do with a lesson he received when he was a young diplomat. He was going through a document, scrutinizing it under the supervision of a senior member of the department, when the supervisor made him go back and attend more precisely to the wording of a particular clause. "Now there," said the man, "is a minor point of major significance."

If there is anything that links diplomacy, artistry and surgery, it is the way they all rely for their success upon attention to minor points of major significance. So I must ask you to allow me to draw attention one more time to the poem about the fiddler on the Blaskets. He had a Pentecostal visitation, all right, and the tune came to him out of a mighty wind, but what distinguished him was his ability to carry it through, to make a job of it and bring it back whole. I can't remember whether O'Riada's original story involved the bit about other fiddlers making their night vigils and not quite managing to piece together the tune because of technical inadequacy; I suspect I may have made it up myself to emphasize the link between wholeness and technical readiness, as it were. At the time I wasn't thinking about W. B. Yeats's poem, "Adam's Curse," where Yeats makes a similar point when he declares: "It's certain there is no fine thing / Since Adam's fall but needs much labouring." Nevertheless, "The Given Note" is among other things a parable about the way the fine thing depends upon the quality of the skill and effort that go into it: "Strange noises were heard / By others who followed, bits of a tune / Coming in on loud weather // Though nothing like melody. / He blamed their fingers and ear / As unpractised, their fiddling easy // For he had gone alone into the island /And brought back the whole thing. / The house throbbed like his full violin."

Another island. Another airspace. Not the Blaskets this time, but somewhere off the map, somewhere brought home to us in Shakespeare's play *The Tempest*. In a famous scene in *The Tempest,* Caliban, the man-monster, the creature described in the *dramatis personae* as a savage and deformed slave, speaks about a tune the characters hear coming out of the clear blue sky. His two companions, you remember, the drunken sailors Stephano and Trinculo, are bewildered by the music—music that's being played, as Trinculo says, "by the picture of Nobody," although the audience knows it is being played by Ariel. "Art thou afeard?" Caliban asks and Stephano answers, "No, monster, not I." And then Caliban speaks the well-known lines:

Be not afeard; the isle is full of noises,
Sounds and sweet airs, that give delight, and hurt not.
Sometimes a thousand twangling instruments
Will hum about mine ears; and sometimes voices

That, if I then had wak'd after long sleep,
Will make me sleep again: and then, in dreaming,
The clouds methought would open, and show riches
Ready to drop upon me; that, when I waked,
I cried to dream again.

This is the story of *port na bpúcai* being told for Shakespeare's audience in the Globe Theatre. Caliban cries because in his daily existence he remains shut out from the beauty and wholeness to which Ariel's spirit music gives momentary access. And in Caliban's cry of longing it is possible to recognize our own. Beauty is transitory, the whole thing comes and goes, life is not solved but there is a momentary sensation of resolution, a healing moment. What Caliban might have said of the music, for example, is what each of us might say of the Shakespearean poetry that describes it: "It did me good."

To put it another way, the do-goodery of poetry and of the arts in general is fleeting and occurs first and foremost as an intimate experience. If it is to have effect, poetry must be felt by the individual, must register, however minimally, on the scale of the personal. Before it can become a shared value and a general force it must be known as an event in an individual's emotional life, be recognised, whether consciously or unconsciously, as an experience that is worthwhile. Poetry begins, as Robert Frost puts it, in delight, before it ends in wisdom. The writing of a poem, he goes on, "runs a course of lucky events, and ends in a clarification of life – not necessarily a great clarification, such as sects and cults are founded on, but in a momentary stay against confusion."

Frost mentions sects and cults in order to distinguish the kind of "clarification," as he calls it, upon which they are based from the kind of "clarification" that a poem can provide. What sects and cults do, of course, is to preach a message, which they want everybody to embrace and to practise as a manifestation of true faith and right conduct. My suspicion is, however, that by "sects and cults" Frost here meant the most widespread and historically established systems of religion, the great world faiths that claim to possess the universal truth. But whatever he meant precisely, there can be no doubt about the general distinction he was insisting on. The poet, Frost is saying, doesn't set out to start a movement or to institutionalise a vision. Whatever good poetry does is done unofficially, as it were, on a one-to-one basis.

Frost's claim, therefore, with which all modern poets and artists would be in agreement, prompts us to raise a question about the general efficacy of poetry: we may be ready to grant that it is in itself a whole and a good thing, but we might want to know how the rightness and goodness of an individual work (and the private experience of it by a particular reader or audience)—how exactly that helps to heal or make whole whatever happens in the world beyond.

People undoubtedly want such an effect and such a carryover to exist. At times of general distress, at times when sects and cults and systems of faith are confident in the proclamation of their doctrines and dogmas, people want the arts to come up with something that will match their needs. When circumstances are at their most bewildering and most overwhelming, people need an articulation that will act as a momentary stay against confusion, yes, but as something more. They want to be brought *beyond* confusion.

Never was this clearer than in the days following the attacks on New York and the Pentagon last September. There was a feeling that a crack had run through the foundations of the world, that the roof was blown off, that the border between the imaginable and the possible had been eradicated. For millions of Americans, danger and terror crossed from the realm of fantasy and nightmare and entered the historical record. A catastrophic event happened in full view of all the nations of the earth. Neither the common mind nor the common language was prepared for it. It was the most widely registered, commonly shared, universally acknowledged wound ever delivered to a *res publica* in peacetime. And yet what could be said? What words could match it?

Religious language sprang naturally to the lips of leaders. Talk of good and evil fulfilled a need and gave an order to the threatening chaos. Stupefying hurt and righteous anger found some expression in absolute terms like good and evil, crime and punishment, war and defeat. All this was designed to bring us beyond confusion but in many minds it had the opposite effect of opening a gap. Many people experienced a misfit between the settled, definite nature of those mighty words and the dismayingly unsettled, indefinite condition into which we had been propelled. Talk of "the first war of the twenty-first century" inevitably brought back memories of the first war of the twentieth. High rhetoric in high places, high certainty about God on our side, high flags, and high patriotism—all this seemed to belong to an older dispensation. It was as if we were suddenly back in the age of righteous militarism and divinely sanctioned aggression, and as a result there occurred what I am calling a misfit: what was happening out there was at variance with what we were inwardly prepared for. But that bewilderment only made the need for an articulation or a figuring of our plight more urgent; we wanted to be able to summon images and formulations from our cultural tradition that might still be capable of establishing our co-ordinates in the new reality.

Listen, for example, to these words, written by a Polish poet in an introduction to a recent anthology of Polish poetry: the

author is Stanislaw Baranczak and his thoughts on the function
of culture in the life of the individual are both clear and cogent.
"As a rule," Baranczak writes, "there is an intermediary between
society's experience and the individual's psyche—a kind of
go-between that can be called culture. If not for that, the
outer world of facts and events and the inner world of language
and feelings and thoughts would resemble two interlocutors
speaking different languages with no way to communicate.
It is precisely culture that serves as an interpreter—an interpreter who helps us to understand what reality tells us and
what it asks us about, and who, at the same time, helps us to
formulate our own questions in a comprehensive language of
symbols. With culture," Baranczak goes on, "perhaps the most
apt interpreter of this kind is poetry."

"A kind of go-between" that relates "the outer world of facts
and events" to "the inner world of language and feelings and
thoughts" by discovering and deploying "a comprehensive
language of symbols"—that is a most satisfying description of
what art and artists, poets and poetry are up to. And that
language of symbols, Baranczak insists, is not just for *reflecting*
the outer world but for helping us to formulate our own
questions to it and about it.

Take the case of Wilfred Owen, for example, the English
poet who in early 1915 answered the call to join up and fight
the Kaiser when more men were needed to act like patriots,
defend the cause and rally to the flag. Owen, like millions of
others at the time, on both the German and the British sides,
was ready to fight and die; honour brought him into the field
and made him a courageous and decorated officer. But horror
at what he saw and at what he had to do made him a poet
with an anthropological as well as an artistic meaning for the
century that followed and for the century we are now entering.
Owen made his own particular contribution to international

health and to the advancement of a braver, newer world when he questioned and put into doubt much that the outer world received and took as normal. At the height of the war fever, when the ranks were closed and the mind shut against doubt, he was bold to ask if it was indeed *dulce et decorum pro patria mori?* In the age of mechanized slaughter, was there still truth in Horace's noble sentiment that it is sweet and honourable to die for one's country? Was there ever truth in it? Owen not only battled the enemy on the front line, but he attacked the enemy of complacency and insensibility on the home front; by going to war, he won the right to speak out against the war, and in the century that followed his death, his poems were of great human value, performing like cultures that grew their own pacific and conscientiously objecting yeasts. I would like, therefore, to let you hear one of Owen's most famous poems, the one called "Strange Meeting," and to say a few words about it, because in it poetry did for Owen in particular exactly what Baranczak says it can do in general: it allowed him to conduct a dialogue between his inner world of language and feelings and the terrible outer world of facts and events that he was living through in the trenches, and it further allowed him to express this dialogue in a comprehensive language of symbols.

The trenches were indeed hell on earth, and it's as if Owen took this colloquial hint and proceeded to elaborate it to the fullest of his emotional and technical ability, using the richest deposits of the civilization he was in the trenches to defend. The hero who descends into the underworld to meet the shades of the dead is an archetypal figure in western literature. He appears in Homer's *Odyssey* when Odysseus goes down into Hades; he reappears in Virgil's *Aeneid* when Aeneas walks among the shades in Avernus; and then the underground journey takes on its specifically Christian and more conventionally hellish connotations in the fourteenth century of our own era when

Dante writes his *Inferno*, the first part of *The Divine Comedy*. In that poem, the pilgrim poet walks among the damned and treats them as the enemy. They have been cast out by God and doomed to punishments that they deserve to suffer for all eternity. No sympathy is required for them, no sympathy is allowed them and no sympathy is given. But in the hell upon earth that the twentieth century soldier-poet inhabits and reinterprets in his inherited language of literary symbols, sympathy is given, blame is removed and enmity is replaced by friendship. The inner man knows that he has been betrayed by the rules of the outer world, and answers back with one of the seminal poems of the past hundred years, one in which Christ's command to love the enemy and do good to them that hurt you is answered in a high style and at a high price.

When he wrote "Strange Meeting" on his last tour of duty, not long before he fell to machine-gun fire in the last week of the war, it was as if Owen went alone into the island and brought back a whole thing. And he was able to do it not only because he was spiritually prepared but also because his fingers and ear were by now well practised. He was ready technically. He had played tunes on his instrument and perfected his skills, in particular the technique of half-rhyme or para-rhyme. And in the circumstances this was the right sound. Instead of perfect chimes like "shaped" and "escaped," or "groaned" and "moaned," Owen employed rhymes that were just a bit off, "scooped" and "escaped" or "groined" and "groaned." The consonants matched perfectly but the vowels were not entirely the same, and in this dissonance, in this particular failure of wholeness, Owen diagnosed the whole failed thing in European society at the time and also made a homeopathic gesture towards its healing. "Strange Meeting" is a poem in which he gave beautiful and grievous expression to what he called elsewhere "the eternal reciprocity of tears."

Strange Meeting

It seemed that out of battle I escaped
Down some profound dull tunnel, long since scooped
Through granites which titanic wars had groined.
Yet also there encumbered sleepers groaned,
Too fast in thought or death to be bestirred.
Then, as I probed them, one sprang up, and stared
With piteous recognition in fixed eyes,
Lifting distressful hands as if to bless.
And by his smile, I knew that sullen hall,
By his dead smile I knew we stood in Hell.
With a thousand pains that vision's face was grained;
Yet no blood reached there from the upper ground,
And no guns thumped, or down the flues made moan.
"Strange friend," I said, "here is no cause to mourn."
"None," said the other, "save the undone years,
The hopelessness. Whatever hope is yours,
Was my life also: I went hunting wild
After the wildest beauty in the world,
Which lies not calm in eyes, or braided hair,
But mocks the steady running of the hour,
And if it grieves, grieves richlier than here.
For by my glee might many men have laughed,
And of my weeping something had been left,
Which must die now, I mean the truth untold,
The pity of war, the pity war distilled.
Now men will go content with what we spoiled.
Or, discontent, boil bloody, and be spilled.
They will be swift with swiftness of the tigress,
None will break ranks, though nations trek from progress.
Courage was mine, and I had mystery,
Wisdom was mine, and I had mastery:
To miss the march of this retreating world

Into vain citadels that are not walled.
Then, when much blood had clogged their chariot-wheels
I would go up and wash them from sweet wells,
Even with truths that lie too deep for taint.
I would have poured my spirit without stint
But not through wounds; not on the cess of war.
Foreheads of men have bled where no wounds were.
I am the enemy you killed, my friend.
I knew you in this dark; for so you frowned
Yesterday through me as you jabbed and killed.
I parried; but my hands were loath and cold.
Let us sleep now....

Let me recap here and then move towards a conclusion. I read "Strange Meeting" because it has often done me good to read it. It has the virtues which I claimed for poetry earlier in the lecture. It is a thing formally and feelingly sound, right in itself, a thing to which the ultimate response is "yes." Something has been brought through and brought home. It is clearly the result of dreamwork, but it could not have been composed without the writer's specialised skills and heightened intuitions being brought deliberately and intensely to bear. If it does not solve the confusions of a person's experience in time of war, it gives at least a momentary sensation of resolution; it is like a slow air that rephrases itself into the air and it has registered so memorably and so tenderly in the consciousness of individual readers that it has long ago entered the store of shared values that we call our culture. And this whole process of one poem's composition and reception and integration into cultural memory is an example of the way poetry helps to promote the wholeness of things in general.

Still, while poetry may indeed promote it, it can by means guarantee such wholeness. For poetry, as I have said in other contexts, is like the immunity system of the spirit; it works for good but it cannot always withstand assault. Or perhaps I might use another image drawn from the world of the healers and say that poetry is a kind of drip feed, and when it works it percolates down out of its own refined element into the common speech and understanding of a whole society.

In a famous set of lines, W. B. Yeats once declared: "The rhetorician would deceive his neighbours, / The sentimentalist himself, while art / Is but a vision of reality." And in another more challenging and slightly mysterious phrase, he talked about his effort "to hold in a single thought reality and justice." And this attempt was made, he said, through "the stylistic arrangement of experience." Such efforts are as concentrated as any other serious, life-focusing, life-committing activity, although they are perhaps less obviously so. The poet in the act of composition may not show the strain the way the man with the pneumatic drill shows it, or, for that matter, the surgeon holding the scalpel. But the *pneu* (as in pneumatic) may be shaking the poet inwardly every bit as much as the drill shakes the worker, because the poet's *pneu* is immediately derived from the Greek word meaning breath or spirit, so it means also an inner excitement and breath of life that parallels the outer movement of the blowing winds.

And there I might well very well end, for we have come full circle, back to the fiddler on the Blaskets, getting his air out of the night. But I want to conclude instead by returning more specifically to the question of the good of poetry, the question of whether it can be said to maintain in any real sense the health of the world; whether it and its practitioners can still fulfil their ancient office and responsibility to sing out and make sense and take the measure of reality.

I want to go back, therefore, to those days after September 11.

I felt called upon to do something that would be an answer, that would be a form of response, because it is precisely by making a written response that a writer exercises responsibility, and a writer's sense of his or her success or failure will often be based on how satisfactorily he or she rises to the challenge of the historical moment. At any rate, during those days of crisis in the inner and outer life I heard no

spirit music on the wind, but then, in a quiet way, a god did speak to me in my attic study on Sandymount Strand Road. I happened to be sorting through the texts of old lectures I gave last year at Harvard and found in one of them a reference to an ode by Horace. At Harvard, I had used this particular ode to conclude a talk about poetic inspiration, and in the course of the talk I discussed Robert Graves's notion that all poems are the gift of a muse whom he called "the white goddess." I had also quoted Graves's poem about this goddess figure, which ends with a line that says he is always ready for her visitation and "Careless of where the next bright bolt may fall."
Then I said:

"We may be shy of going the whole way with Graves, in the over-the-topness of his Muse worship, but we know that poetry can never afford to renege entirely on its covenant with the irrational. It comes along to shake the usual into an awareness of its own precariousness. Its bright bolts are like the ones I read about in the thirty-fourth ode of Horace's First Book of Odes where Jupiter hurls his thunderbolts without warning into the blue of an Italian afternoon."

And when I came upon those words, I knew that I simply had to translate Horace's poem because it is, in the fullest sense of the word, tremendous. It is about *terra tremens,* the opposite of *terra firma.* About the tremor that runs down to earth's foundations when thunder is heard and about the tremor of fear that shakes the very being of the individual who hears it. In the poem, Horace expresses the shock he feels when the thunder-god drives his chariot across a clear blue sky: usually, the poet implies, he would be ready for thunder and lightning because usually there would be a massing of clouds and a general sense of threat in the atmosphere. This time, however, the god had arrived so suddenly there was no time to prepare for his terrific sound and fury, and it almost seemed that the safety of the world itself had been put into question. The poem is in four stanzas, the most powerful of which are the two in the middle: these possess an uncanny strength and sooth-saying force and give the whole first century BC scenario an eerie contemporary applicability. I realise, of course, not everyone will understand the Latin original, but it is still worth hearing:

Parcus deorum cultor et infrequens
insanientis dum sapientiae
consultus erro, nunc retrorsum
vela dare atque iterare cursus

cogor relictos. Namque Diespiter,
igni corusco nubila dividens
plerumque, per purum tonantis
egit equos volucremque currum;

quo bruta tellus et vaga flumina,
quo Styx et invisi horrida Taenari
sedes Atlanteusque finis
concutitur. Valet ima summis

mutare et insignem attenuat deus,
obscura promens; hinc apicem rapax

Fortuna cum stridore acuto
sustulit, hic posuisse gaudet.

A literal translation may also be useful. This one is in prose and is a slightly updated version of an 1887 Victorian rendering. Its very datedness is probably useful in that it keeps the poem (for the moment) at a certain cultural distance:

"I have been a reluctant and infrequent worshipper of the gods, have steered my own course and gone with the usual madness, but now I am forced back on myself, compelled to turn my sails, and retrace the course I had forsaken:

For the Father of the sky, who mostly cleaves the clouds with a gleaming flash, has driven through the undimmed firmament his thundering steeds and flying car; whereby the ponderous earth and wandering streams are rocked, and the Styx and grisly site of hateful Taenarus, and the limits of the sea where Atlas stands.

To change the highest for the lowest, the god has power; he makes mean the man of high estate, bringing what is hidden into light: Fortune, like a predator, flaps up and bears away the crest from one, then sets it down with relish on another."

Obviously, there was an eerie correspondence between words "valet ima summis mutare….deus" (the god has power to change the highest things to/for the lowest) and the dreamy, deadly images of the Twin Towers of the World Trade Centre being struck and then crumbling out of sight; and there was an equally unnerving fit between the conventional wisdom of the Latin "obscura promens" (bringing the disregarded to notice) and the *realpolitik* of the terrorist assault, in that the irruption of death into the Manhattan morning produced not only world-darkening grief for the multitudes of victims' families and friends, but it also had the intended effect of bringing to new prominence the plight of the Palestinians.

Still, the original is a poem of religious awe, not a political comment or a coded response to events. It is the voice of an individual in shock at what can happen in the world, and there and then it came to me that the phrase "Anything can happen" would be a fair twenty-first century translation of the Latin "valet….deus" (a/the god is capable) and that it would also give specific voice to the reality of the world in the autumn of 2001.

Once I had taken this liberty, I was emboldened to take more, and ended up with a version in which the whole first stanza is dropped, and "rapax Fortuna," the predatory goddess at the end, becomes an image of the impulse to attack or to retaliate, whether that impulse be unleashed or repressed. But I believe the translation still does justice to the sense and emotional import of the original while operating as a fair enough answer to what has happened in our own present time. I called it "Horatian Stanzas."

Anything can happen. You know how Jupiter
Will mostly wait for clouds to gather head
Before he hurls the lightning? Well, just now,
He galloped his thunder-cart and his horses

Across a clear blue sky. It shook the earth
And the clogged underearth, the River Styx,
The winding streams, the Atlantic shore itself.
Anything can happen, the tallest things

Be overturned, those in high places daunted

And the ignored regarded. Fortune wheels
And swoops, making the air gasp, tearing off
Crests for sport, letting them drop wherever.

As I said at the start, previous lecturers in this series have been people whose contributions to the good of the world have been practical: peacemakers, healers, researchers, and campaigners. I have tried to argue that poets have rights in this company because there is good in finding words that allow the inner world of language and feelings to connect with the outer world of facts and happenings; words that stay firm when we press upon them, that won't let us down when we ask them to take the strain of reality, words that have been brought back as a whole and healing gift by those who went alone into the island of themselves and their world.

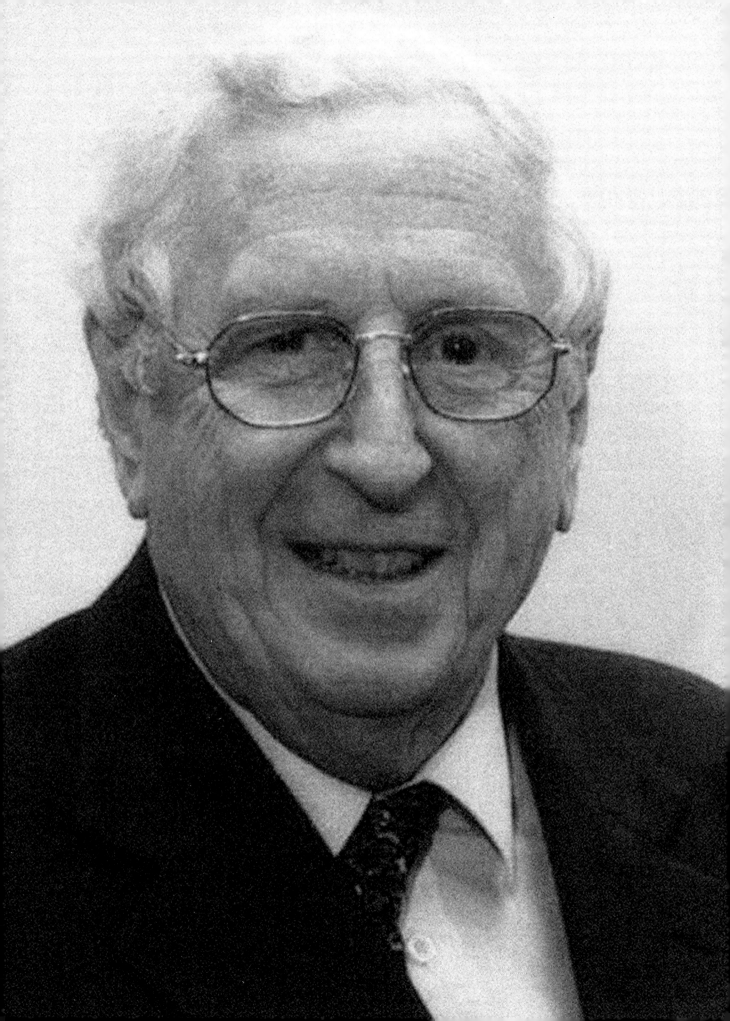

Garret FitzGerald

His Distinguished International Lecture was delivered in the College on October 26, 2000.

Garret FitzGerald was twice elected Taoiseach (Prime Minister) of Ireland. He had been Foreign Minister, and his efforts in both positions led towards the Anglo-Irish Agreement in 1985, the first official step on the path to peace in Northern Ireland. In addition to his political achievements he had a long career as an academic, author, journalist, and columnist. He worked for Aer Lingus for many years, taught economics and political science, and eventually served as the Chancellor of the National University of Ireland. One of my many fond memories of this remarkably modest and humble man was having dinners in their home when he was Taoiseach; because his wife, Joan, was wheelchair bound and could not climb stairs, they had moved to the basement suite in their house in Dublin. There the Prime Minister would not only greet you, but cook and serve the meal, and then clean the dishes afterwards. Garret died, a much beloved man by friends and countrymen, in 2011.

The Unique Instability of Irish Demography
Garret FitzGerald

Why am I talking to you tonight about demography?

Well, the first answer is, of course, that I choose the subject myself simply because I felt like talking about it!

But this is a subject which should concern doctors amongst others—and I think I'm safe in assuming that there are quite a few doctors here tonight—because medical people are by definition concerned about both births and deaths—whatever about marriage! And births and deaths, together with the movements of people, are fundamentally the matters I shall be talking about—because it is these that govern all shifts in population.

Demography is about people: Such matters as how many are born, how long they live, whether they stay put, or migrate elsewhere. Economic growth rates are in significant measure a function of population growth or decline. The truth is that, of its very nature, demography lies behind everything to do with people.

Now, we happen to live in a country which over the past couple of centuries has had one of the most unstable demographics in the world—with more ups and downs, and twists and turns, than, I believe, any other. At various points we have in demographic terms been the leastest—and then again the mostest: we are above all a land of demographic extremes! And this fact goes a long way towards explaining many odd things about this country.

Let me list a few of these demographic extremes.

First of all, it is sometimes forgotten that just one hundred and sixty years ago Ireland was one of the most densely populated parts of what is now the European Union: its population density was then almost twice the European average of that period. Only Belgium and a couple of Italian city states had a higher population density than ours.

(Where did I get EU figures for the 1840's? Happily I have a number of copies of the Almanach de Gotha, stretching back over 200 years. This was the key European reference work from the late 18th century onwards, from which the subjects of monarchs could find out all about their rules and their rulers' families and genealogies—but also details of governments, of diplomats, of populations and of the physical extend of Europe's 45 states of that era. Every house should have one!)

Today, 160 years later, our population density, from having been twice the EU average, is only two-fifths of that average. And from having had, 160 years ago, one-twenty-fifth of the population of the area now comprised by the EU, we now have only one-hundredth of the Union's population—viz. 1%.

Let me give you another example of Irish demographic extremes. Before the Famine Irish people married young. However, after that tragic event, late marriage became the norm; indeed until the middle of the last century one-quarter of those born never married.

However, with economic growth in the 1960's, all that changed. And by 1971 the initial stage of our economic expansion had created a quite new situation, where half of all women were marrying by the age of 24. Moreover before long the proportion never marrying had fallen to less than one-tenth.

In terms of the ratio of marriages to the number of women aged 20 to 34, the marriage rate peaked in that year—just three decades ago. But shortly afterwards came a third turn-around. From the mid-1970's onwards the marriage rate, measured in terms of the young female population, began to fall again. During the ensuing quarter of a century it dropped to less than half its 1971 peak level—until, in late 1995, it started rising once again! Since then the ratio of marriages to younger women has in fact increased by about one-tenth.

So, since the 1840's—which to me at least is not so very long ago, three of my four grandparents having been born in that decade, whilst in my childhood I met several people born around that time—since then we have had no less than four absolute reversals of our marriage rate!

Now let me give you yet another tale of demographic ups and downs.

Between the 1880's and 1930's the proportion of non-marital births in Ireland more than doubled to 4%. However, by the mid-1960's it had more than halved again to a record low of 1.5%. But since then this proportion of non-marital births has risen more than twenty-fold, to 33% today. And over half of all first pregnancies today are non-marital—three out of every eight of these pregnancies being aborted in Britain—something quite inconceivable a generation ago.

Yet another radical demographic shift has, of course, been the fall in infant mortality, which during the last War temporarily rose to over 10% in Dublin. Today, at barely one-half of one per cent, our infantile mortality rate is, of course, among the lowest in the world—as is the death rate arising from pregnancy—now less than two per year, and none at all in some years, as against well over 200 annually sixty years ago.

And, associated with the infantile birth rate, yet another turn-around. We are inclined to forget – if we ever knew! – that up to the mid-1930's, which is a decade after my generation appeared on the scene, one in six of all those born was dead by the age of 35. For, of those who survived infancy, many died of TB in their teens or twenties.

But just thirty years later, for the age cohort born in the mid-1960's, the pre-35 death rate had fallen from one out of six to one out of thirty.

As for migration, up to the 1950's we were losing over one-third of our young people to emigration. When this attrition was added to the high death rate of that period amongst young people, the result was that less than half of those born here survived in this country to age 35. That's a kind of third world statistic – although death rather than emigration is the prime decimator of those populations.

This deeply depressing picture was all changed by the economic growth that we began to achieve in the 1960's. Throughout the 1970's we actually enjoyed net immigration – as we are again doing today.

During the 70's some 25,000 former emigrants of the male sex returning to work here – almost all of them accompanied by a wife, and an average of two children – thus giving us a net inflow of 100,000 over that ten-year period.

But then came the economic disaster of the late 1970's – which I had the bad luck to inherit as Taoiseach, and to have to tackle. By the year 1986 the resultant astronomic inflation had been brought under control, a huge external payments deficit had been eliminated, unproductive capital spending had been cut, the borrowing rate that had faced us in 1981 had been halved – and the task of getting our finances in order was completed by Ray McSharry between 1987 and 1989.

(I am, of course, aware of the continued adverse impact even today of the cuts in the health service which he imposed in those years: no doubt he could have handled that part of his work with more finesse. But the economy as a whole certainly benefited from his brief term of office).

But the human cost ultimately imposed by the financial mismanagement of the years before 1981 was huge. Within a six-year period in the 1980's net emigration had once again cost us over 200.000 young people – although some 50,000 of these have since found it possible to return here.

Let's just take today's cohort aged 30-34 – that is, the 310,000 people who were born here between 1964 and 1969, and follow their fate. By 1981 that age group had been swollen by over 25,000 children brought back to Ireland by their parents, returning home during the years since 1969.

However, during the following decade well over one-quarter of that whole age cohort – that is, some 90,000 young people in their twenties – had been forced to emigrate in search of a job. And that figure must have included some thousands of those who as children had been brought to Ireland by parents returning to work here in the 1070's.

However, within the past nine years over 25,000 of that 90,000 have returned here again – and several thousand of these have thus returned for the second time to the country to which they had first been brought as children!

I frankly wonder whether there is any other country in the world that has had such an extraordinary history of flows of young people backwards and forwards, of the kind we have experienced during the past three decades. Somehow, I doubt it! Please excuse this shower of figures. I have just been trying to justify my initial statement that Irish demography has been uniquely unstable. And I think I have done that!

This little understood fact has had important consequences for public policy in Ireland – the significance of which is not always understood here – let alone anywhere else!

Some of these consequences are quite widely known and quite well understood, e.g. the fact that our population will soon be starting to age, and – a matter of major concern to the medical profession – the fact that life expectancies are low in Ireland, for reasons that certainly include life-style factor, as well, perhaps, as deficiencies in our provision for certain forms of disease.

I don't intend to dwell on these fairly well-rehearsed issues – beyond commenting that, whatever about our low life expectancy, where much needs to be done, we are relatively well-placed in respect of the aging and pensions issue.

On the one hand that crisis is going to hit us much later than other European peoples, because of a combination of the high rate of attrition of past generations by early deaths and emigration and the fact that our birth rate peaked later than anywhere else in our continent. The problem will not start to emerge in any perceptible way for another decade or so and will not peak until around 2035.

Moreover we are currently making a better start at providing for this problem by setting aside 1% of our GNP annually so as to build up a fund out of which to supplement future pension payments from current resources.

Instead I am going to say something about two consequences of demographic change that have attracted too little attention: the impact of demographic factors upon the future growth of our labour force, and important changes that have been taking place in the pattern of Irish births.

Demography and the Labour Market

Part of the good side of our demographic turmoil has been the fact that because our birth rate peaked in 1980, which was several decades later than in the rest of Europe, recently we have been enabled to increase our work-force very rapidly.

For, because of this fact, the flow of young people from our educational system into our work-force has for some time past been adding to employment here at a rate half as great again as in the rest of Europe.

Unfortunately much of this bonus is now about to disappear - because between 1980 and 1995 our birth rate fell by over one-third. The impact of the bulk of that decline is going to hit us during the next seven years – reducing by almost 30% the potential third level entrance cohort.

With unemployment now down to 3.5%, the drying-up of this important component of the annual renewal of our labour force – the flow of young people from our education system into the labour market – is bound to have effects upon our economic growth rate.

For three-fifths of that growth has in fact come about through increasing employment – more people at work – the remaining two-fifths being the outcome of improvements in productivity.

There are, of course, two other sources of extra workers in addition to school-leavers and the unemployed, viz. the movement of women from work at home to paid work, and immigration.

But both of these are also going to come under pressure in the years ahead.

Already our employment participation rate for women in their 20's is the highest in Europe, so in order to increase female employment further we now have to depend largely upon the return to work of older women – those who in earlier decades left the labour force to undertake child care. Over time, as the work participation rate of these older age groups grows, this must inevitably become a diminishing source of new labour supply.

As for immigrant workers, the inflow of such workers has already added to our housing demand on a scale that must account for a good deal of the huge pressure on house prices here. And that rise in house prices is beginning to slow the growth of this type of immigration.

Changes in these four demographic factors affecting our work-force are not going to choke off our economic growth overnight. But we certainly cannot go on expanding our economy by 8% a year for much longer. And if the Government does not face this reality fairly soon, we are in for a lot more inflation than the price of oil is currently accounting for!

A by-product of the growing shortage of labour has been the emergence since 1996 of a premature movement of boys out of the educational system. Less boys are continuing in education after Junior Certificate; less are continuing to higher education; less are undertaking higher degrees. The educational level of our male population, which rose rapidly from the late 1960's to the mid-1990's, looks like taking a dip henceforth – to the long-term disadvantage both of those concerned and also of our economy.

This development, which has not yet started to affect the female half of our young population, also has potential implications for the already rapidly shifting relationship of the two sexes to each other.

Changes in our Birth Pattern

Let me mention one other recent demographic change that also has important implications for the future of our society. The decline in our birth rate was reversed in 1995: the number of babies born here in 1998 was one-tenth greater than in 1994 – and right into the current year this increased birth rate has been maintained.

This is partly because there are now quite a number of births to asylum-seeking women, who, as an unintended by-product of the Belfast Agreement of 1998, now have a right to remain here if they become mothers.

But the principal cause of this increase in births has been the continuing rapid rise in the number of non-marital births, the number of which has jumped in this five-year period by as much as two-thirds, to one-third of all births.

This recent period has also seen a continuation of the rise in the average age of mothers at birth. To some extent this has reflected the fact that, not just recently but throughout the whole of the past two decades, the growth in non-marital births has been accompanied by a rise in the proportion of such births that are to mothers aged 25 or over. Non-marital births are no longer a teen-age or young twenties phenomenon, for there has been a growth of longer-term non-marital unions, within the framework of which a minority of couples are now content to procreate and bring up children.

But the principal factor pushing up the average ago of mothers at birth during the past two decades has in fact been postponement of marriage, and the associated postponement at the age at which married women have their first child. Twenty years ago, i.e. around the time that our birth rate peaked, barely one eighth of first marital births were to wives aged 30 or over. By last year this proportion had almost trebled to well over one-third.

When later births are taken into account, 55% of all births are now to women aged over thirty. Twenty years ago, when larger families were three or four times more common than to-day, the proportion of babies born to women over 30 was only 40%. At that time with the help of contraception very many women were completing their families by the time they reached their early thirties, whereas today many women of that age are only starting to have children.

Mainly as a result of later marriage, the decline in the number of births to women aged 40 and over, which had dropped from over 8% of all births in the mid 1960's to 3.25% in the mid 1990's, has now halted. And the proportion of births to women in their late thirties has been rising quite sharply during the second half of the last decade.

This reflects the fact that, from having been the European country where the proportion of women at work was lowest and where women married youngest, we have moved almost overnight to being the European country with the highest proportion of younger women engaged in paid work – and thus with latest age of marriage and highest age for births.

In this as in so many other respects we are not only the country of greatest demographic extremes: we are also the country that has moved fastest from one extreme to the other.

Sudden drastic changes in demographic behaviour often tend to impose great strains on society, and it is clear that our society is at present suffering from a number of strains of this kind. There are two observations I would make about this.

One the one hand our system of government has been notably slow to recognize, never mind to react to and seek to cushion such changes.

But on the other hand these often-dramatic social changes, affecting the family in all its forms, have created much less inter-generational tension than might reasonably have been expected. Humanly we have coped well with the fastest and most dramatic demographic and social revolution any European society has experienced. And that's just as well, in view of our inveterate institutional sluggishness!

I leave you with that thought!

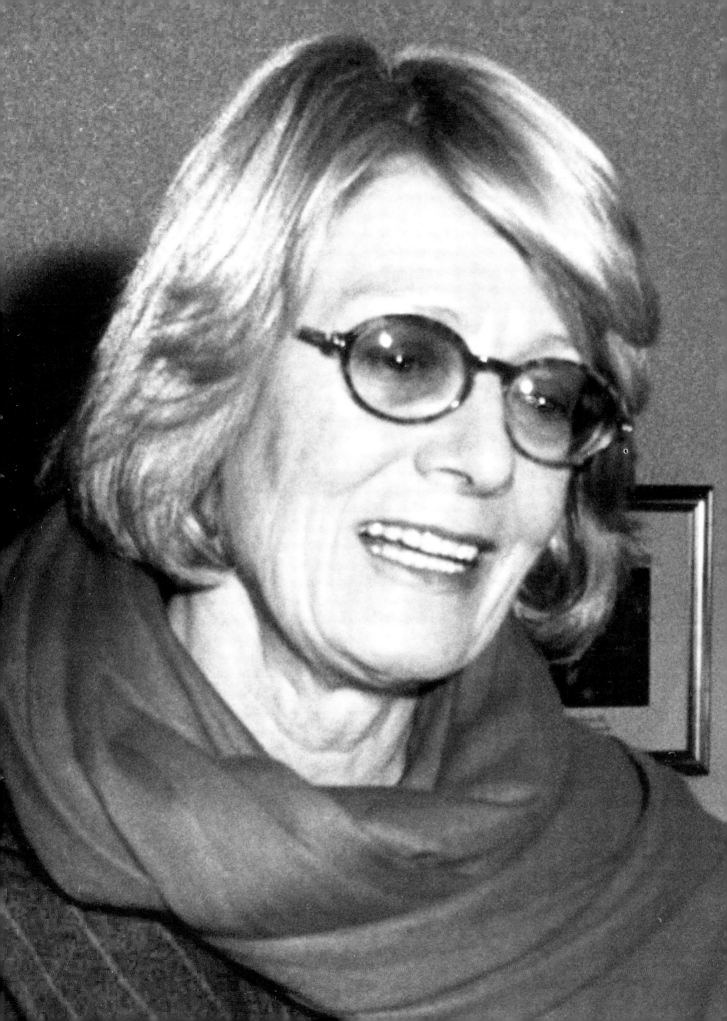

Vanessa Redgrave

*Her Distinguished International Lecture was delivered
in the College on November 1, 1999.*

Vanessa Redgrave was born into a family
which had worked in theater, and later also
in cinema, since the 1880s. She made her
stage debut in weekly repertory, graduating
to work in Shakespeare at Stratford on Avon,
and with contemporary English and American
playwrights. She has been honored with the chief
British and American theater awards, five
Oscar nominations, an Emmy and many
international Film Festival Awards.
She has used her skills and talents and passion
to focus attention on the rights and needs of
families and children and to raise funds and
support for them in emergencies. She has
been a UNICEF UK Special Representative since
1991, and a UNICEF Goodwill Ambassador
since 1995. I have been privileged to
collaborate with her, and her family, on many
humanitarian projects.

Keeping a Promise
to My Albanian Friends
Vanessa Redgrave

When I gave a talk at the Royal College of Surgeons in Dublin on November 1st 1999, at the invitation of Professor Cahill, I was very tired, and also, as the transcript of my talk proves to me, very incoherent! So when Kevin asked me to edit the transcript, although I said "yes" because who could say no to Kevin when he has always said "yes," I did hesitate.

I have checked back on a recent letter from Prishtina, dated August 6, 2013, from my friend, the producer/director and actor Fatos Berisha:

"Dear Vanessa, We haven't been in touch for some time. I hope everything is fine on your side. Meanwhile, here in our little country (its been 5 years of independence) things are pretty much the same. For me, I was working for two years for the Kosovo Film Center and now I feel time to go back to the festival; this year will be the 5th year since I was one of the founders of the Festival, and you are our Honorary President…As you can remember, we invited you last year, wanting to honour you with Honorary Golden Goddess for your contribution to Kosovo's culture and film community. You were busy that time, but what are the chances to come this year?"

Fatos emailed me again on September 3rd, explaining his drive to set up a Foundation to help young filmmakers in Kosovo and the region. A co-production Forum at the Film Festival in Prishtina where filmmakers from Kosovo, Serbia, Montenegro, Macedonia and Albania can pitch their film projects has been part of the Festival for the last four years. As I was due to open a new Shakespeare production at the Old Vic four days later, sadly, I could not accept to attend the Prishtina International Film Festival this year. I had attended the first festival in 2008, ten years after my very first journey to Kosovo in 1998 during what is known on Wikipedia as the Kosovo War.

In 2003, I had filmed in Zagreb and other locations in Croatia, "The Fever" directed by my son Carlo Nero, and televised by HBO Films. In 2006, my sister Lynn and I, and Amanda Plummer had performed a project, rehearsed on Brijuni island in Croatia, and then performed on Goli Otok, the island off the Croatian coast where Tito's women political prisoners laboured, were tortured, and died in the 50s and 60s. This performance, titled "Core Sample" incorporated scenes from Beckett's "Waiting For Godot", music by composer Nigel Osborne, and monologues we had transcribed from interviews with some women survivors of "Goli Otok." The production was part of ULYSSES annual theatre festival produced and directed by my dearest friends Rade Serbedzia and his wife Lenka Udovicki. I invested 100,000 dollars in this production, and Rade and Lenka's ULYSSES Theatre Festival. I have returned to Sarajevo to sing with Rade in concert, and also to Belgrade and to Llublyana in Slovenia. All of this since the Dayton agreement of 1995, when the first peacetime Sarajevo Film Festival began with an open-air screening of "Mission Impossible" in which I appeared with Tom Cruise. In 2009, I had filmed in Belgrade, playing Volumnia with Ralph Fiennes for his "Coriolanus."

Why should I write this down? Because Rade and Lenka, and their friends, have been my inspiration since I first met them in Manchester, England, in 1993, when they and their baby daughter, were both basically refugees from Belgrade, with a small temporary home in Slovenia, and a good friend, English actor Antony Andrews. And why do I think it might be worth the while of anyone to read a little of what I tried to explain about Kosovo in November 1999, at the Royal College of Surgeons in Dublin?

In the late 1930s my father Michael Redgrave joined a small number of English actors, in trying to get British visas for performing artists and film makers who were attempting to escape Hitler's Nazi regime which was occupying more and more of Europe. To get visas was made intolerably difficult by the Chamberlain government. Those who know the story of the great Austrian artist Oskar Kokoscka, know how hard it was for him to obtain a visa to come to Britain. Walter Lassally, the lighting cameraman, was one of the filmmakers who finally got a visa. Martin Miller, a German actor obtained a visa, and my father along with others gave him money regularly so he could have some accommodation and food once he arrived, for he was destitute.

In September 1939, when Britain finally declared war on Nazi Germany all the London theatres closed. Then, they re-opened for a while, even as heavy bombing began, when the Government ordered them closed again. My father went as part of a delegation to a Government Minister requesting to reopen the theatres and concert halls of London for lunchtime and afternoon performances. He knew that theatre, concerts and films were essential if people's spirits of resistance were to be maintained.

I was reminded of this when I first went to Sarajevo, for UNICEF, in 1993, and many times after during the terrible siege by the Serbian armed forces. It was the Bosnian theatre and music professionals who kept the spirit of resistance to cold, hunger and death throughout the siege. It was they who played for children in basements. It was they who rehearsed through bombing and sniping so youngsters could have classes in drama, painting and singing. I rehearsed and performed there in 1994, and this time I was able to enlist the enthusiastic support of a wonderful UNESCO lady to obtain the permits for the Haris Pasovic theatre company to fly out of Sarajevo to perform in Paris at Peter Brook's theatre, and afterwards return.

Human Rights and Humanitarian Aid are too often misused for various governments' political agendas. Nevertheless, doctors and nurses, paediatricians and counsellors, and teachers step up to the plate, as Kevin Cahill did when I asked him to medically examine an Albanian Kosovar girl asylum seeker whom I had found in a prison in New York. The actors, filmmakers and musicians, who I have come to know since 1993, are the ones who can keep the spirits and hope alive, whether of children or adults. As a driver in Kosovo said to me in September 1999, "The soul needs food as well as the body."

Wars have passed, leaving bereft families, and a bereft culture of many youngsters, deprived of access to the production and entertainment of films and plays, and rock concerts, and football, and classical music.

The filmmakers, musicians and theatre people who became my friends in Kosovo work with their ever-growing numbers of friends in Serbia, Croatia, in Montenegro, and Macedonia and in Slovenia. This has been going on for some years. What assistance are they getting? Sponsors are hard to find, governments have small budgets and many urgent demands. The European Union did not fulfil their promises. Real estate and property investment have eager seekers and promoters.

The fact is that the new refugees of today are the re-builders for tomorrow. The artists in theatre, film, TV and music and dance are the lifeline, in each country, and across the frontiers, from the past through today and on.

On a dark, rainy autumn day in 1998 I drove with an Albanian Kosovar actor from Skopje to Prishtina. Over nine days I drove with him, or a young Albanian journalist from "Kohaditore", or with Flaka Suroi who was the regional officer for UNICEF, in and out of Prishtina, to Peja (Pec in the Serbian language) over hills, through devastated villages and ruined homes, meeting families sheltered under plastic tents, small schools in tents, women and children who had seen their husbands and fathers beaten and shot in front of their eyes. I talked with human rights lawyers, and filmed them. I saw their meticulous files and photographs of battered bodies and cut throats. I met the chief doctor heading the Mother Theresa Society on whose assistance some 500,000 jobless and homeless Albanian Kosovars depended. I met actors and theatre directors and drama students, and musicians. The doctors and nurses of this brave Society were categorised as terrorists by the Serbian authorities; arrested, jailed, beaten, or murdered on the spot.

When the Serbian army and police, and the paramilitaries forced tens of thousands of Albanians including my friends at gun point out of Kosovo into Macedonia in 1999, I returned to Skopje and to Tetovo to find them. I raised money to help them. We gave performances for children at the giant refugee camp of Cegrane on a flat bed truck loaned from UNHCR. Mark Brooking, a relief worker with CARE, sucked petrol from a container to fuel the generator for the microphones! When NATO forced a way open for the withdrawal of Serbian tanks and armed forces, other friends were murdered by Serbian paramilitaries. When it became clear that the way was now open for the refugees to return to Kosovo, we began to make plans for a Festival of Music to commemorate The Return.

It became clear we must begin in Skopje, and proceed to Prishtina. I suggested that the concert in Skopje should commemorate the terrible earthquake of many years before. This was needed to overcome much tension in Macedonia, where the police had beaten the refugees when they were forced into this country. Besides many Albanians lived in Skopje, and Tetovo, and the Macedonian government had allowed a semi-official Albanian language theatre, a vital relic from Tito's Brotherhood and Unity days.

I had to do some filming in Canada, and there I met Philip Glass and a miners' choir in Nova Scotia. I then approached the Canadian Minister for Foreign Affairs for funding for a three day concert. I received his call pledging finance as I hid behind a bush on a Halifax seashore, about to film a scene! Philip Glass stayed true to his word and brought Foday Musa Suso to join him for the Skopje concert, which was a sell-out that September. I made countless journeys into Prishtina, had countless meetings with my colleagues, who included Fatos Berisha, and countless meetings with the UN organisations. Bernard Kouchner said he had a problem he could not solve. Once I found out what the problem was this was easy to solve. I asked my friend, British theatre producer Bill Kenwright, to be the official producer of these concerts, in association with me. Bill was entitled legally to insure the concerts, and he came to the plate in every way magnificently. He brought Lulu, and a rock band to Prishtina. Lulu of course was the delight of the British Army whom I had approached for a brass band to play for us. Jack Lang, the French Minister of Culture brought a very famous French singer from France. My husband, actor Franco Nero, helped me to win the support of Maria Pia Fanfani and the Italian Carabinieri. I pitched in money and brought four dancers from the Martha Graham company, thanks to Ron Protas, Martha's former personal assistant. I also brought my dear friend concert pianist Katharina Wolpe, and my eighty-eight year old mother Rachel. Of course many Albanian singers and musicians played and sang over the two days, which ended with the Canadian miners and their lamps marching into the indoor football stadium where some 10,000 youngsters applauded them. They greeted my mother with such shouts and cheers that not a word she spoke from Chekov's *Uncle Vanya* could be heard.

There were some very sad and dark moments before and after. For example, I visited the parents of Adriana, a drama student I had met in 1998. She had been shot and killed by police in the café where she and other student friends met after a class with Enver Petrovci, the actor and director. One of the leading human rights lawyers had been murdered as he left his offices, where Serbian police destroyed all the files and photographs. My film on cassette had been rendered unusable.

I end with homage to Nexhmija Pagarusha. I met this elderly lady, who was still known by Albanian Kosovars as the "Nightingale of Kosovo" when we sat together for the first time in 1998 in a Prishtina café. As a teenager in 1945, after the Second World War she sang every week on Radio Prishtina. Her five-octave voice enchanted everyone. Then In 1974 President Tito inaugurated the period known as the Brotherhood and Unity time. Festivals were held in all the Republics of Yugoslavia (Kosovo was never granted the status of a Republic). The singing contests usually ended with prizes in Belgrade; Nexhmija won 1st, 2nd or 3rd prizes every year; "The Belgrade media, the journalists who reported on radio and in the newspapers had no idea what language I was singing in. They would ask if I was singing in the Macedonian language if they asked at all. They thought Kosovo was perhaps a small village in Macedonia. And Milosevic continues to proclaim that Kosovo is the heart of Serbia!"

When you have the good fortune as I have had, to make good friends and work with them, and listen to them, you can understand so much more clearly what the media and the politicians don't see, and never seem to grasp until much much too late. As for re-building a country after war, and re-building infrastructure on which life depends, that is a specific story. A human story, the European Union has largely neglected. Even Paddy Ashdown was unable to get the funds for Bosnia, so desperately required, when he was High Commissioner there. I have tried to give a brief idea of the role of theatre, music, and filmmakers and performers in re-building the arts facilities in their countries.

I raise my cap to Kevin Cahill whose expertise, dedicated work, and inquiring eyes and ears and mind has raised the education of international humanitarian aid efforts to a new level.

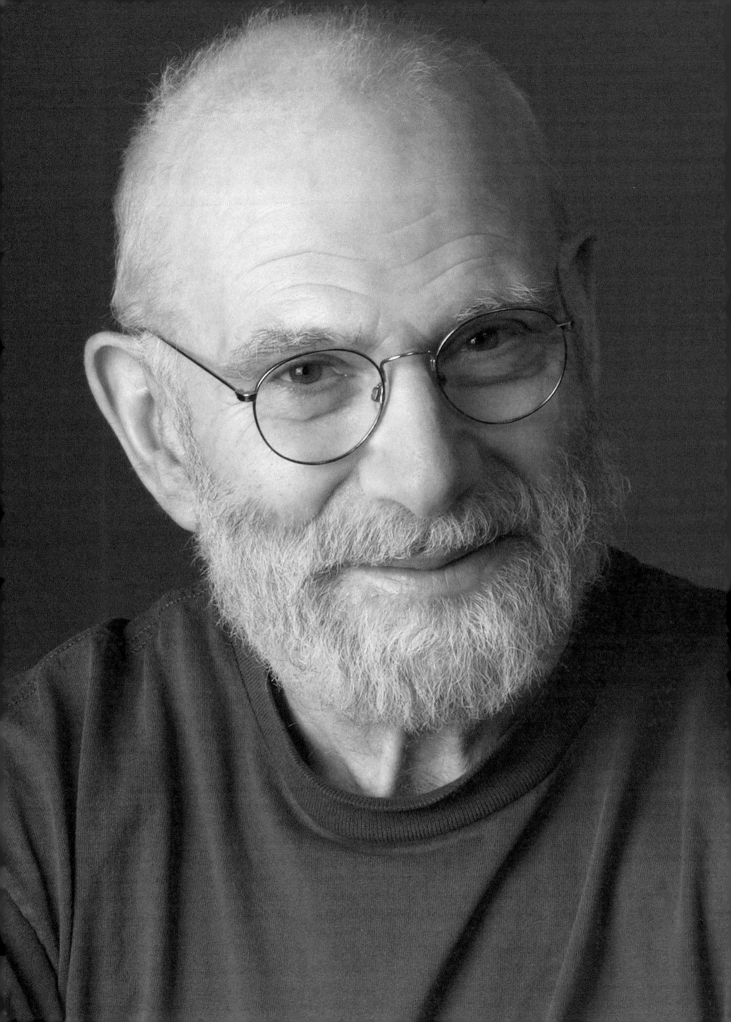

Oliver Sacks

His Distinguished International Lecture was delivered in the College on October 29, 1998.

Oliver Sacks, M.D., is a physician and writer whose interest in the links between body and mind, and the ways in which the whole person adapts to different neurological conditions, has won him an international following. He received his medical degree from Oxford, and is currently Clinical Professor of Neurology at New York University. He wrote a classic medical text on *Migraine*, but is best known for his books for the general public on the far borderlands of neurological experience. *Awakenings, The Man Who Mistook His Wife for a Hat, An Anthropologist on Mars,* and *The Island of the Colorblind* have all been best sellers. The New York Times has referred to him as "the poet laureate of medicine." He has also books about, *inter alia,* ferns, musicophilia, and chemical elements.
He has an asteroid named in his honor! I have had the inordinate privilege of sharing long conversations, ocean swims, concerts, and complex clinical cases with Oliver over many decades.

Neurology and the Soul
Oliver Sacks

It's exciting to be in Ireland again and a very special pleasure being here at the Royal College of Surgeons in Dublin. I feel honoured and happy (and slightly bewildered!) to find myself part of this series.

I have used the word "soul" in my title because it seems to me a much more powerful word than "identity" or "self" or anything like this. The word "soul" gives one a sense of something alive, growing, evolving, multiform, manifold and almost infinitely deep, and with a sort of centre; and I think a concept of this sort is necessary in neurology and psychology, and goes beyond the Freudian concept of the ego. So if I speak of soul I don't mean anything infused or immortal, but I do mean the fullness of a person – biological, cultural, personal, spiritual – and I want to speak of its survival, its adaptations and vicissitudes, in the context of various neurological disorders or damage.

Osler used to say "Ask not what disease the person has, but rather what person the disease has." This is going to be a central part of my theme. It is essential to get a narrative, a personal narrative, of how a disease is experienced by an individual, the particularity of the impact. A mere pathography is not enough. Medicine requires one to elicit symptoms and signs, and from this to arrive at a diagnosis, and then to embark on some sort of treatment. But I think this is only the beginning, and although someone may have, for example, a migraine – a clear and physiologically-defined condition – the migraine occurs in the context of a particular life, the unique pattern and economy of a life, and if you are to understand it you need to look beyond the bare diagnosis, to get a sort of biography from the person. So getting stories and telling stories, putting stories together, seems to me to lie at the very heart of clinical medicine.

One might be concerned at the notion of medicine being reduced to clinical algorithms, of medical judgement being replaced by expert systems. One needs, of course, to have some knowledge and skill, and to think logically and strategically, but all this has got to be embedded in an imaginative projection as to what is actually going on with a person. One cannot be a physician without imagination and empathy, without an intense effort to imagine oneself in another's position.

Forty years ago, when I was a medical student in London, my professor suggested that I see a new patient who had come in. He said "Go and see the delirium in bed six," in much the same way as surgeons sometimes speak of "the appendix in bed eight." My professor added, "He is dying of uraemia...he is delirious. Spend a few minutes with him, see what a delirium is like." I spent more than a few minutes. I spent hours, I spent days, I spent all my spare time for a month listening to this man in his delirium. And in his delirium he brought out memories of events and scenes and people he had known, of passions and hopes and thoughts he had experienced. An entire life, an entire soul came out in the broken, hieroglyphic form of delirium. It was very remarkable, like being privy to a dream. So this was not just a delirium. It was his delirium—and his whole life, his perspectives, his identity, his soul were clearly there, behind the myriad disconnections in his brain. This gave me a strong feeling of the robustness of identity, and even in a sense its indestructibility, despite very severe and diffuse brain pathology. This is a theme I may return to, if I get to speaking about Alzheimer's disease later.

I mentioned migraine before. I was newly emerged from a neurological residency and tended to think very physiologically when, in 1966, I saw a patient, a young man who had "sick headaches" every Sunday. He gave me more details, described the scintillating zigzags he had before the headache, so it was easy to make the diagnosis. I said "You are having migraines," and that we had specific medications for this, and if he put this ergotamine tablet under his tongue as soon as he saw the zigzags, this might serve to abort the attack. He phoned me up in great excitement the following Sunday. He said the zigzags had started, but he had put a tablet under the tongue and — wonderful, miraculous! — there was no sick headache. He said "God bless you doctor!" and I thought "Isn't medicine easy?"

The next Sunday I didn't get a phone call and I was curious as to what might have happened, so I phoned him up. This time he told me in a rather tired voice, the tablet had worked, he hadn't had a migraine — but, he complained, he had been profoundly bored. He didn't know what to do with himself. Every Sunday for the previous fifteen years had been devoted to migraines; his family would come, he would be the centre of attention — and now he missed all of this. The Sunday after this I got an emergency phone call from his sister saying that he was having a severe attack of asthma, a veritable status asthmaticus, and there was a suggestion in her voice that it was perhaps my fault, that I had "rocked the boat." When I saw my patient later that day he said that as a child he had indeed had attacks of asthma which had later, apparently, been "replaced" by migraine, and he wondered whether, now that I had "deprived" him of this, he was going back to the asthmas again! I told him we could treat the asthma, but his reaction was strange: he nodded his head and said something which seemed to me rather extraordinary.

He said, "Do you think I need to be ill on Sundays?" Having had a narrowly physiological sort of orientation in my residency, I was taken aback, but I said, "Let's discuss it," and we then spent two months (avoiding medication) exploring his putative "need" to be ill on Sundays. As we discussed this, his migraines got less and less intrusive, and finally more or less disappeared—all without any medication. So for me this was an example of how, sometimes, one cannot abstract an ailment, or its treatment, from the whole pattern, the context, the economy of someone's life.

Another patient comes into my mind, who also had migraines on Sunday—these "sabbatical" migraines are not uncommon, and they often tend to occur in rather driven, obsessive people who relax over the weekend. [I am told that such migraines tend to occur in priests on Mondays, but in the rest of us on Saturdays or Sundays.] This man, a mathematician, would have one of these fierce Sunday migraines, and then, in its resolution, a lysis—a pouring out of various secretions, diuresis, diarrhoea, diaphoresis, etc.—a sort of catharsis in a physiological way, followed by an access of creativity and good feeling, almost a re-animation. This would carry him through a halcyon Monday and Tuesday when he felt the most creative mathematically; then, on Wednesday, he would feel a little tense, not able to concentrate so well, and on Thursday and Friday he would be even tenser, become agitated, and, finally, have a migraine again on Sunday. This was his cycle and had been for years.

He responded to medication in a way both therapeutic and disastrous: it cured his migraine but it cured his mathematics too! His creativity and his migraines seemed to be linked, and it seemed somehow impossible to treat one without affecting the other.

I want to speak now of another encounter – the "Awakenings" experience which Professor Cahill referred to. When I first went to Beth Abraham Hospital in the Bronx in 1966, I encountered nearly eighty patients in the corridors and the lobby, some of whom were "transfixed" and petrified in strange attitudes. I had never seen patients like this. I had seen catatonic people on the back wards, but this was different, and I was amazed and awed when I heard that some of these patients had been like this for thirty or forty years, and indeed that the hospital had been opened in 1920 for these first victims of the epidemic sleepy sickness. I at first wondered whether these people had anything inside, whether there was any inner life, or whether they were as inanimate or de-animated as they at first seemed to be, but the nurses, many of whom had been at the hospital for decades, were convinced that there were intact minds and personalities in these patients; they also mentioned that there were occasional, very brief "liberations" – these might come with music, for example, when patients who could not walk might dance, and speechless ones sing; that in music there might be (in the few minutes it lasted) a relief, a freedom and fluency, an emergence of self and soul, which was otherwise buried in their frozen, catatonic states.

But one couldn't make any long-term change until the medication L-dopa came along. One knew that L-dopa was very useful in ordinary Parkinson's disease, of fairly short duration. These people had a much more complex illness. Many of them had been violently hyperactive, sometimes manic or frenetic or full of tics, in the early days, although this had then been submerged by the parkinsonian catatonia. Von Economo, who described the whole course of the illness, spoke of such patients as having become "extinct volcanoes," but I thought that they might be dormant volcanoes instead; and what if one were to "uncap" them and remove the constraint of parkinsonism, what then might happen?

And then there was an existential problem of an unprecedented sort. These were people who in some sense had come to a stop, physiologically, psychologically, decades before, and had been put away, often abandoned, removed from the world. Where were they? If one could get them going again, where would they be? In this context I thought very much of something which James Joyce wrote about his daughter who had gone mad: "Fervently as I desire her cure," he wrote, "I ask myself what then will happen when and if she finally withdraws her regard from the lightning-lit reverie of her clairvoyance, and turns it upon that battered cabman's face, the world." I wasn't sure that there had ever been any precedent; myths like the Sleeping Beauty and Rip Van Winkle went through my mind. I think that in medicine one very often, surprisingly often, meets such intersections of myth and fact.

I hesitated a good deal. I hesitated for two years before doing anything. I tried to obtain consent, but in a way this is paradoxical, because you are asking people to consent to something unimaginable—this is a point I will bring up later in regard to giving sight to people who have never seen. One of my patients once referred to dopamine as "resurrectamine," and when one gave L-dopa there was, indeed, a sort of resurrection which at first was purely delightful and lyrical, but which then proved to be full of paradox and anomaly and difficulty. But the real task, the deepest task, came later and especially had to do with the unprecedented challenge to identity or soul, with these people who had come to a stop decades before.

There was one woman, a very bright woman—I call her "Rose" in *Awakenings*. When she came to in 1969, she started talking and singing constantly. She talked about Gershwin as if he were still alive. She talked a great deal about the 1920s, but always in the present tense. Her talk and her manner and her mannerisms were those of a "flapper" who had come to life. I wondered if she was disoriented, where she thought she was. So I quizzed her, and she said, "I know it's 1969 but I feel it's 1926. I know I'm sixty-four, but I feel I'm twenty-one;" and she indicated that although there had been occasional flash like memories (she had heard of Kennedy's assassination, she had heard of Pearl Harbor, etc.), she had no sense of having had any coherent life or autobiography in the intervening forty-three years. She had dropped, as through a vacuum, from her twenties to her sixties, from the 1920s to the 1960s. Could there be a life for her now, in her sixties, the 1960s? She complained that everything which had had meaning for her had vanished, she said that she didn't like "our" world and after ten days of her strange, twentyish animation, she went back into the remote catatonic state she had been in for forty years, and nothing we could do ever budged it again.

But with the majority of patients it was possible to help them construct or re construct a life or an identity, a world, a self of some sort, despite the enormous discontinuity of their lives. We all need love and work and meaning and relationships and hope and faith, but one saw this in the most extreme way with these patients, and only to the extent that they could construct a meaningful life were they able to tolerate and profit from the continued use of the drug. So here again, but in an infinitely more complex way, one saw that a purely physiological approach was not enough. One had to address the whole person, all the uniquenesses of their souls and lives.

As one continued L-dopa, some of these patients moved from transfixedness to hyper activity, and in some cases to having multiple tics and lunges and blurtings out of words—a state somewhat similar to that of Tourette's syndrome, as it is called—and my own interest in Tourette's syndrome started at this time. I first saw a patient with actual Tourette's syndrome (rather than post-encephalitic "Tourettism") in 1971; but the day after seeing him, I saw three people on the street in New York with it, and the day after that another two, and the day after that another two—I am sure that you can see the same in Dublin. I wondered why I had not recognized these people before. They didn't suddenly emerge one day, they were obviously there all the while. It's very striking—this business of recognition. The novel has to be experienced and categorized in the mind, there has to be a single, striking impact, before one can recognize, or even "see" it again. It was this way with muscular dystrophy, the very severe congenital form which was first described by Duchenne in 1858. Within two years, hundreds of further cases had been described, and Charcot asked how could it be that something which was clearly common, and ubiquitous, and had always existed, was only now being recognized. He said, "Why did we need Monsieur Duchenne to open our eyes?"

A colleague of mine has written a very nice book about Tourette's syndrome entitled *A Mind of Its Own*. Unlike parkinsonism, which is in some sense an automatism, below the level of feeling or intention, Tourette's syndrome often contains a strange sort of intentionality. It can accelerate thinking and association. It can energize one in a sort of way, and it can almost form a sort of personality in its own right. I had one patient who wrote to me saying that he had a "Tourettized soul." I don't think one can have a parkinsonized soul, but one can have a Tourettized soul, a soul in part shaped by one's Tourette's (and a Tourette's in part shaped by one's soul). Tourette's may be manifest and florid by the age of four or five, and perhaps its primordia may occur in the cradle, so in some sense people with Tourette's have grown up with it. It has been their companion all their life, and a very complex and intimate sort of coupling or "siamesing" can occur between the Tourette's and the self.

Given this close sort of coupling, the medical situation and the existential situation become unusually complex. I had one patient—the one who called himself "Witty Ticcy Ray," and was given, in his own words, to "ticcy witticisms" and "witty ticcicisms"—who was a very good amateur jazz musician and who related this, in part, to his Tourette's: he was famous for his improvisations, and some of these would start with a compulsive or convulsive hitting of the drums which would then be rapidly elaborated into a half-creative, half-Tourettic musical furor. When one gave him a medication for his Tourette's, he lost all sorts of troubling tics and impulses, but he also lost his ability to be a creative jazz drummer—a very heavy cost to bear. He finally dealt with this by taking the medication from Monday to Friday, and then he would be calm and sober and unimpulsive in a way which was suitable for his daily work. But over the weekends he would take himself off it, and would get into a sort of frenetic-Tourettic-dionysiac state which was ideal for his jazz extemporizations. Almost thirty years later, he still maintains this balance, and his children realize that their father has two identities—his Monday-to-Friday identity, and his weekend identity. He has two identities, but they are both his. Two identities in one soul, so to speak.

I sometimes want to call Tourette's a brilliant disease because it can energize and drive, but this energizing and driving can, of course, be very destructive. What is crucial is the positive use or employment which some people can make of their Tourette's, the balance which can exist between it and them. Speaking here in the Royal College of Surgeons, I should mention that I not only wrote a story, a clinical study, about a Tourettic surgeon, but that I have now seen nine Tourettic surgeons! I also know quite a number of Tourettic athletes and artists, and many of them have learned to use their strange energies, their impulsiveness, and the often-heightened sensibilities of Tourette's, in highly productive ways. So the question of whether to treat Tourette's becomes a complex one. In general children with Tourette's are treated because these are decisions made by their parents or their doctors or their teachers. Adults with Tourette's may sometimes take themselves off medication and say "Let me be. Let me be Tourettic. Let me be myself." It is especially this question of autonomy and intervention which so needs to be discussed.

Some years ago I got a completely unexpected letter–but medicine consists of unexpectednesses–from a man, an artist, a rather famous artist in his sixties, who told me that three weeks earlier, following a car accident and head injury, he had become suddenly totally colourblind. He had had some other problems, at first–he was unable to read, due to a visual alexia, but the ability to read came back in two or three days, whereas the perception of colour did not. He gave me a vivid description, when I saw him, of how he had driven to work to his studio the next day. He knew it was a bright and sunny day, but it seemed overcast and grey and nebulous. He was stopped by the police, who told him he had been through a couple of red lights. He said he had not seen any red lights. When he got to his studio–his studio which was hung with brilliantly coloured paintings–he found them stark, black-and-white, evacuated of colour, and since colour had been a crucial vehicle for meaning and feeling and organization and expression, his art seemed to have gone meaningless, completely dead, on him. He was terrified at this, and terrified, too, that he might be going completely blind. He rushed back to his wife for reassurance, but this was not reassuring because she had changed (as he put it) into "an animated grey statue." And when he looked at himself he now realized that his own skin was lacking in colour, was grey, and when he closed his eyes to conjure up colour—to try to imagine or remember it—it didn't work. He didn't know what was going on. He didn't know if he had had a stroke, or if, perhaps, he was hysterical. He went to a hypnotist, and was given some sodium amytal—this can sometimes "de-repress" affects or memories, and lead to a sudden "catharsis," and disappearance of hysterical symptoms—but this didn't help, so he came to me.

As a neurologist I could say, "You have sustained bilateral damage in the prestriate areas of the visual cortex, areas necessary for the 'construction' of colour." If one has damage in these areas, one not only loses the ability to perceive colour, but the ability to imagine it, to remember it, to dream in it, the whole lot. I said I didn't know what degree of recovery he could expect, nor anything one might do to improve the chances, but I hoped that (even if there was no neurological recovery) he would find a way of adapting, of living a full life nevertheless. We spoke of making a life, being creative, even in the absence of colour. At this point he had become almost suicidal. He felt it was the end of him as an artist, and the end of him as a human being, and he had been annoyed by people saying "So you have lost colour, big deal, so what?" But for him it was an enormous deal. I think it would probably be for any of us. We take colour for granted. We may admire black-and-white photos or films but that is quite different; and although Mr. I, my patient, first compared his vision to black-and-white television he later said that felt that it was not like this at all, but like being trapped in a world "moulded in lead," and he created a simulacrum of this leaden world in his studio.

But then, about two or three weeks later, he had a singular experience. He was driving to work again (not that he could really work at this time), he was driving out of habit to his studio, rather earlier than usual, and he caught the sunrise. He saw red as black. There was this enormous black sun, this almost apocalyptic sunrise, resembling (he said later) an immense nuclear explosion. He wondered whether anyone in the history of the world had ever seen a sunrise in such a way before. Excited, and inspired, for the first time since his accident, he went and created his first painting in many weeks – he called it "Nuclear Sunrise" – and with this he started to recover his "balance," his interest in the world, his morale, his sensibilities. He did not recover colour, but the colourless world which had been so abnormal and impoverished and ugly now seemed to him to regain an interest and beauty, indeed to gain a new interest and beauty, one that it had never had before. He even felt, in some ways, that his vision had become "more refined," that he was perhaps now attuned to the real "visual essence" of things – contour, brightness, contrast, movement – in a way which had been somehow camouflaged by colour. He earned golden (perhaps I should say silver) opinions when he had an exhibit some months afterwards, and everyone spoke of the old man, the artist, as having entered a most remarkable, creative, black-and-white "period." Very few people realized there had been a neurological disaster – an achromatopsia – behind this creative period. But my point is, the disability had been transformed, had become a sensibility, a most profound and extraordinary transformation. The awful time for him was that intervening time when he had lost one world, the world of colour and familiarity, and had not been able to acquire, to appropriate, the world back in other terms; when one world, one self, had died, and another was not yet born. The terrifying state in which so much support and insight is needed is precisely this limbo between worlds, between losing one world and regaining it, or creating another; and it is especially the ability to construct, or reconstruct, other worlds, other selves, which lies at the heart of "adaptation," and can be so astonishing psychologically, culturally, physiologically, every way. One wonders, sometimes, whether there are any limits to it...

You can see such adaptations, most dramatically, in people born deaf, especially if they are native signers, for from the age of two or three such deaf signers show heightened forms of visual perception, increased peripheral vision, increased ability to parse very rapid and complex movements in the visual field, etc.; and if you examine the brain by electro-physiological methods or brainscans, you find that what would be auditory cortex, what would be the hearing part of the brain, has been "reallocated" for seeing, for visual processing. This business of other senses being keener when one is lost—this is not just anecdotal—there is strong physiological evidence for this.

About three years after his loss a notion came up which we discussed with our colourblind painter, Mr. I, a notion that it might be possible to give him back some colour vision by training other brain areas near the destroyed ones to make use of the visual information which was coming in. He still had the cones in his eye, he still had his primary visual cortex. Whether or not this was possible, what was fascinating was his reaction to our suggestion. He said "If you had offered me this within a few weeks of my loss I would have embraced you. It was what I most wanted. Now I'm not interested. My world has been reconstructed. I have forgotten what colour is like. You can keep it." I found this very strange, I could hardly believe it, but I think it showed (unless he was deceiving himself) the depth of his adaptation, how radically everything else had changed and improved for him. One had to wonder what the physiological basis for this might be, what reorganizations of functions and priorities might have occurred in his brain.

After seeing him I started to wonder what it might be like never to have seen colour, and also at this time my interest was spreading from seeing affected individuals to seeing affected communities. This came together a few years ago when I was able to visit a tiny atoll in the Pacific, where a large minority of the population are born without any cones in their eyes, and therefore without any ability to see colour. Retinal achromatopsia (as this is called) is very rare – only about one in fifty thousand people, in the general community, have it – but in small islands, where there is much isolation and intermarriage, such rare genetic recessives can be greatly concentrated. Thus, in this little atoll of Pingelap, a large number of people (about ten percent of the population) were born without colour vision. When I heard of this I was immediately reminded of an H.G. Wells story (which perhaps some of you have read) called *The Country of the Blind.* This tells the story of a lost traveller who blunders into an isolated valley in South America. He is puzzled by the houses – they are "parti-coloured" – he thinks the people who built these must have been "as blind as bats," and soon he finds this is indeed the case, that he has blundered into a community of the blind, a community who lost their sight so many centuries, so many generations, before, that they now have no cultural memory of ever having seen, and no concept of sight. He imagines that as a sighted man he is superior to them, and can take over. But of course when night comes he stumbles over everything, while they (perfectly adapted to their environment) move around without difficulty. So the tables are turned and now they see him as disabled and demented, and indeed subject to hallucinations produced by these mobile pathologies in his face (which for some reason he is pleased to call "eyes"). He falls in love with a girl in the village and wants to marry her, and when the elders consult, their decision is that they will let him stay only if he consents to the removal of these "eyes," so that he can become "normal" like the rest of them.

It is very interesting and important and humbling and edifying to find oneself in a minority. When we—so-called "colour-normals"—were surrounded by people with no colour vision, in the little atoll of Pingelap, it was obvious that they regarded us as abnormal. They regarded us as obsessed with something non-existent and (they could only imagine) trivial. A ridiculous amount of our attention and language (so far as they were concerned) was devoted to this; they felt we were missing the realness and beauty of the visual world, because we kept jabbering about "colour" all the time, and paid insufficient attention to movement or brightness or texture—for them, the very essence of the visual world.

I spoke to one of them rather insistently saying "How would you like colour vision? What do you imagine it would be like?" After a while he grew tired of telling me that my questions were meaningless, that he couldn't imagine what I was talking about, and he said to me "How would you like X-ray vision?" I thought about it for a few seconds and said "No thank you, I'm fine as I am." He smiled and said "So am I."

Yesterday, in The Times, there was an article about giving sight to the blind, by the use of artificial retinas. Now if one has once had sight and lost it one thinks of it, one yearns for it, desperately, for it has been so central and significant a part of one's life. But if one has never seen, it is another matter entirely, and the question of what might happen if one were "given" sight becomes highly problematic and ambiguous. The possibility of this situation was discussed in the 17th century by the Irish philosopher William Molyneux, who wrote to his brother-philosopher John Locke wondering whether a congenitally blind person who could recognize a glass, a globe, a cube by touch, would be able to recognize it visually if given sight. This was a philosophical question with some personal importance because Molyneux's own wife had, in fact, been born blind. In answer—and there was considerable philosophical discussion—Locke said he thought that the newly sighted person would not recognize anything, but Leibniz (who favoured innate ideas) thought they would. A triangle was a triangle, Liebniz implied, whether it was a visual triangle, or a tactile one. An answer to the question came as early as 1728, when a surgeon, William Cheselden, "couched" the cataracts of a fifteen year old boy born blind; following surgery, the boy indeed saw—saw everything—but, in a bizarre way, he recognized nothing. And this was the situation, the paradox, of a patient I was called to see, a blind man of 50 submitted to a similar operation.

He later gave me an astounding description of how it was when the bandages were first removed. It was expected that he would either say "Hallelujah, I can see!" as in the biblical miracles, or that the surgery would completely fail. In fact what happened was much more complex. There was a long unfocused minute, and it was only when the surgeon said "Well?," that the patient turned toward him, seemed to look at him, in a bewildered "half-blind" way. He himself said that, when the bandages were taken off, he had seen movement and colour—but it was a "pandemonium," unintelligible, shocking. He had thought "My God, is this what they call 'seeing'?" He knew that voices came from faces so, when the surgeon spoke, he turned towards him, but saw only a shifting chaos of planes and colours. He thought "This is a face?" [There was no carryover of the tactile concept of face.] Thus, he saw, but he did not perceive; he was thrown into that state of profound visual confusion, of inability to make visual recognitions, which neurologists call "agnosia." In an earlier book I wrote about a man who mistook his wife for a hat. A man who saw everything, but could recognize nothing. In his case this was due to the destruction of certain associative areas in the visual cortex. In the case of the blind man given sight, it was because these areas had never developed in the first place. The first weeks and months of life are crucial for seeing. You have to learn to see. You have to correlate size and distance and perspective. You have to correlate seeing with the other senses. This is an immense task performed unconsciously and automatically in the first weeks and months of life, and it is necessary for the visual brain to develop. This had not happened with this man. Arduously and consciously after the surgery he tried to do what should have occurred, would have occurred, unproblematically, automatically, in infancy.

In fact, the first time I saw him, there was a strange sort of scene. He had the cat on his lap and he was examining it bit by bit. He would feel an ear, feel the tail, feel a foot, and then look at it. I said "What are you doing?"

He said "I am correlating the cat." It was very difficult for him. It was in some ways an adventure, but in other ways a disaster. Crossing the road had been easy for him as a blind man, but became a new terror and a danger now he was sighted but agnosic, unable to judge objects, or size, or speed. He knew how to function as a blind man, but as a sighted, agnosic man he could hardly function. He became very depressed and he spoke of the gift of sight as "a curse." This has happened in almost every case since 1728. There hadn't been much discussion of possible consequences before the surgery, but one wonders, as with the *Awakenings* patients, what "discussion" in such a context could have been like. How can you say to someone who has no concept of seeing, "How would you feel about having sight? Will you permit us to give you sight?" So in some sense here, as with so many of the patients I have mentioned (going back to the man with the sabbatical migraines), it turned out to be morally and medically problematic, inconceivably complex, to intervene without looking at the whole life situation, and from the point of view of the patient.

Now obviously (and speaking here in the College of Surgeons) I am not against intervention. I wouldn't be standing here myself had good surgeons not done crucial surgery on both my legs. Once, when I was working in a nursing home, I heard an awful choking sound; it was a man having a seizure who, in a convulsive inspiration, had drawn a chicken leg into his windpipe. He was a very bad colour when I saw him, and obviously one couldn't do any of the usual manoeuvres, one could only do an on-the-spot tracheotomy with whatever lay at hand (in this case a steak knife). It had been twenty years since my Anatomy days, I didn't know if I would cut his throat, but luck was with me and I did the tracheotomy okay. There was a deep gasp, and he came to. I am not against intervention. I will intervene as decisively as the next man if need be. But in these complex cases of chronic and lifelong illness, and even with something like migraine, one must enquire into the total experience of illness, its impact, the whole physical and psychical economy of the person. You must look at their entire lives, and not only their personal lives but the whole context, all the cultural aspects too. For example, if a deaf person is an intimate member of the deaf community using sign language he may feel that he would be exiled from his community were he to be given hearing. It is not just a personal decision, it is a cultural decision, too.

Identity, Personality, Soul, whatever you want to call it, starts to develop as soon as the ovum starts to develop. It is sculpted in all sorts of ways by one's life experiences, one's language, one's relationships, one's culture. At this level, people are not even physiologically the same. At this level, Irish physiology is different from English physiology, or Micronesian physiology, and your physiology is different from mine. At the highest levels, we are all unique individuals, souls, and our individuality is embodied in our nervous systems obstinately, faithfully, even in the face of very advanced disease. Even with something like Alzheimer's disease or with deliria one is oneself until very late—when Henry James had a terminal pneumonia delirium, it was said that his ravings were, not only Jamesian, but "late James" in style. Style, character, is the deepest thing in our being. After having been a doctor for forty years, it seems to me that the words of Osler about not just looking at the disease the person has, but at the person the disease has, are the wisest and deepest in the world. I pray there will never be a medicine which is purely mechanical, or which divorces itself from individuality, or the soul.

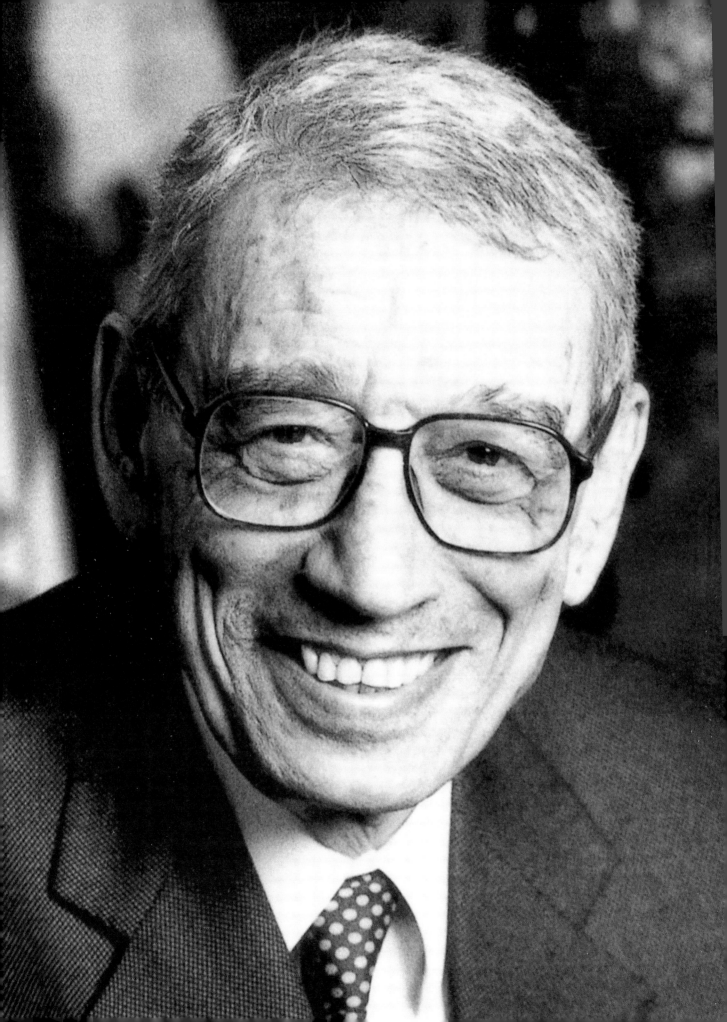

Boutros-Boutros Ghali

His Distinguished International Lecture was delivered in the College on September 22, 1997.

Boutros Boutros-Ghali was the sixth Secretary-General of the United Nations. He was the first Arab and the first African elected as leader of the world body. During his tenure, he oversaw crises in the Former Yugoslavia and Rwanda and authored *An Agenda For Peace*, a document that provided for a more robust role for U.N. peacekeeping missions. Prior to his election at the U.N., he had been Deputy Prime Minister and Minister of Foreign Affairs in the Republic of Egypt; he was a Professor of International Law at the University of Cairo and has lectured on international affairs in numerous universities around the world. After completing his tenure as U.N. Secretary General, he served as the President of *La Francophonie*, the global association of all French speaking nations. He is currently the President of the Academy of International Law in the Hague, and Honorary President of the Human Rights Commission in Egypt.

Peace-Keeping in the Post Cold-War Era: Peace Development and Democratization
Boutros-Boutros Ghali

My dear friend, and physician, Professor Cahill, ladies and gentlemen. It might be appropriate in these ancient medical halls to note that, in my experience, preventing the malady of conflict may be even more difficult than preventing the diseases that afflict the mind and body of human beings.

There are no guaranteed vaccinations to prevent conflicts from starting and no miracle cures to end them once they have started. The best prevention is for the region or country concerned to follow a strict and healthy regimen of democratization, human rights, equitable development, confidence-building measures, and respect for international law, while eschewing indulgence in such unhealthy practices as nationalism, fanaticism, demagoguery, excessive armament, and aggressive behaviour. Most of the elements of such a regimen are prescribed in the United Nations Charter and in the corpus of international law.

The difficulties of prevention in the field of peace and security do not arise because the warning signs of conflict are more difficult to detect than those of human disease; on the contrary, they are usually more obvious. Nor is it that the therapies are less effective; many effective therapies have been devised over the years. The United Nations dispensary is well stocked and many experienced consultants and specialists are on call.

The problem is with the patients and with the friends and enemies of the patients. Human beings may be full of phobias and superstition about disease but they can usually be relied upon to respond fairly rationally to the diagnoses and prescriptions of their physicians. The same cannot, alas, be said of governments and other parties to political conflicts. Many general practitioners would have been tempted to retire in despair long ago if their advice had been disregarded by their patients as consistently as the advice of the United Nations is disregarded by those to whom it prescribes therapies to avert imminent conflict. But the Secretary-General of the United Nations cannot abandon his principal duty any more than a conscientious physician can abandon a difficult case. The Secretary-General's duty is to use all the means available to him, be they political, military, economic, social, or humanitarian, to help the peoples and governments of the United Nations to achieve the goal, emblazoned in the first paragraph of its Charter, of saving succeeding generations from the scourge of war.

Peace-keeping in the post-Cold War era is a comprehensive problem covering three main fields, Peace, Development and Democratization. These must be our focus. All three are interlocked and I will try to explain what this means by acting on the 3 agendas I presented during my mandate as the Secretary-General of the United Nations: *Agenda for Peace 1992*, *Agenda for Development 1994* and *Agenda for Democratization 1996*.

Peace-keeping, development and democracy are being redefined and extended in the post-Cold War era. The connections between them are beginning to emerge. We will need a new level of understanding, and a new depth of commitment to understand the importance of this connection.

Let me mention each in turn. The first concept is Peace.

I. Peace

With the heavy hand of ideology lifted, violence erupts in many regions of the world. The United Nations in the Cold War decades created the concept of peace-keeping. After the Cold War the United Nations peace-keepers took on vast new duties. The United Nations started as many new operations in my term as Secretary-General as in the previous 45 years. Peace-keeping costs for 1993 exceeded $3 billion, more than three times any previous annual figure. There were 18,000 peace-keepers, out numbering the armed forces of almost 75% of its Member States. In the eight years from 1986 to 1993 the annual cost of peace-keeping to the United Nations increased more than twelvefold from $234 million to over $3 billion, without counting the peace-keeping costs borne directly by the countries that contributed troops to those operations.

We must realize that today's operations are not "peace-keeping" in the traditional sense. Those earlier missions involved United Nations' forces which were lightly armed. Firstly, they were interposed between two States in order to maintain a cease-fire. Secondly, they were there with the agreement of all concerned. Thirdly, they were an international presence, not a force expected to take drastic action or to intervene.

Today, United Nations operations may take place, in the first instance, where there is no peace to keep. Secondly, they take place where new forms of assertive action may be required. United Nations forces protect relief shipments, provide services for victims, respond to refugee needs, enforce embargoes, remove personnel mines and seek to confiscate arms. Thirdly, United Nations operations now involve a large civilian dimension beyond military-related steps, such as monitoring elections, public safety, information and communication, institution-building, and the restoration of infrastructure and administrative services.

Peace-keeping today is vastly different from the past in both quantity and quality. It is even chronologically different. Peace requires preventive diplomacy, peace-making, peace-keeping and post-conflict peace-building. The cycle continues through perpetual rounds. Increasingly, we can see that work for peace provides us with no place of rest. It is a continuous process. Peace-keeping must take place: before, during, and after conflicts.

1) *Before conflict*, preventive diplomacy is of vast importance. In matters of peace and security, as in medicine prevention is self-evidently better than cure. It saves lives and money and it forestalls suffering. This approach has traditionally involved personal contacts, good offices, fact-finding missions and early-warning systems. No other endeavour for peace repays our time, effort and investment so well.

Today, the concept of preventive diplomacy is expanding. Your own Professor in this College, Professor Cahill, has been an international leader in this field. It may require for example, observers as a means of dealing with violence. United Nations observers in South Africa, in Haiti, in Georgia and Guatemala have helped reduce tensions, contain demonstrations and stop clashes from getting out of control.

And within this concept has come a step never before taken by the United Nations: preventive deployment. In December 1992, the Security Council decided to put units of United Nations peace-keepers into the former Yugoslav Republic of Macedonia, in order to deter a wider Balkan war. This is an example of the new range of actions needed for preventive diplomacy in the future.

2) *During conflicts*, expanded forms of peace keeping are taking place. In a growing number of conflicts, protection of

humanitarian relief shipments is required. This need was most dramatically evident in Somalia. Similarly, the Security Council authorized United Nations forces to secure the Sarajevo airport and related lines of communication so that vital humanitarian aid could get through in the former Yugoslavia.

Enlarged peace-keeping during conflict also may require sanctions when cease-fire agreements break down. Military measures such as "no-fly" zones may be involved. In Cambodia, in 1992, the Security Council imposed petroleum sanctions against any party not complying with the cease-fire disarmament or national reconciliation requirements of the Paris Agreements. And when the rules of engagement for peace-keeping operations are not sufficient, United Nations forces may need authorization to react to force. In some cases, they may use force to prevent an escalation in violence. In the former Yugoslavia, for example, in Eastern Slavonia, if territory was not given up in accordance with an agreed peace plan, "peace enforcement" by United Nations troops on the ground was the only solution.

3) *After conflicts* must come post-conflict peace-building. This involves sustained efforts to identify and support structures to build trust and well-being among peoples. Such measures including commercial, cultural and educational projects which are necessary to build bridges between parties to a conflict. The goal is to forestall a re-emergence of cultural and national tensions which could spark renewed hostilities. Without such efforts, no peace agreement is likely to last for long. The concept of post-conflict peace-building is the counterpart of preventive diplomacy, which seeks to avoid the breakdown of peaceful conditions. On a deeper level, both are contributions to the second stage of work for world peace: development.

II. Development

Just as the concept "peace-keeping" needs a new definition, so it must be for the concept "development." What was once a matter of economics is now seen to involve many other dimensions.

We are forced to this new perception by the failure of development as it has been known. The Soviet model for development has collapsed. Western policies and programs of assistance have often proved disappointing. Development, in its traditional meaning, has failed to transform poor countries and countries in post-conflict situations. Achieving a new foundation may well be the most difficult intellectual task of our time.

The situation is however, far from hopeless. There is no excuse for pessimism. It is true that many socio-economic problems have not been solved. But it is also true that many countries have radically transformed their societies and economies. Industrialization and information technology provide a new basis for co-operative international progress. And this has contributed to agreement on some common values and a shared vision of the kind of world we want to see: the global villages of tomorrow.

Development cannot guarantee peace, but without development on the widest scale, we know that the young will be restless and resentful. Land will not be productive. People will fight for resources. And creativity will be misdirected and disorder may prevail.

Without a new and workable concept of development, the United Nations will face an endless sequence of conflicts of the sort we are confronting at this moment. And new conflicts, with worsening implications, can be expected.

Like peace keeping, development is best understood as a matter of stages.

1) ***Before conflict,*** development can help prevent conflict from breaking out. By engaging people's energies positively, development can absorb the impact of differences, can ease confrontations and can help avoid economic and social deterioration.

2) ***During conflict***, development is replaced by humanitarian relief. Under conditions of conflict, development cannot go forward. Instead, it is replaced by humanitarian relief and assistance to people made hungry, driven from their homes or otherwise harmed by the fighting. Such relief efforts, even when successful, conclude with a situation that is worse than before conflict began.

3) ***After conflict***, development takes the form of reconstruction. When conflict has stopped, true development once again has a chance to take root. Post-conflict peace-building can start.

A long-term vision is required at this point. An example is the new concept of sustainable development. At Rio in 1992, the leaders of the Member States of the United Nations agreed that every nations domestic economic policy must take into account its impact on the global environment. In this way, the Rio Conference added to the body of established principles that bind us all. Abuse of the environment for economic gain subverts its very purpose; it kills the goose that lays the golden egg. Sustainable development will be central to development's new definition.
In 1995, which was the fiftieth anniversary of the founding of the United Nations, a Summit on Social Development took place. It has provided a new momentum in favour of the concept of development. It calls upon us to produce a comprehensive vision and an integral plan of action. It was the moment when all the many dimensions of development were brought together.
The third concept is democracy.

III. Democratization

There can be no flowering of development as I have described it without the third great theme I want to emphasize: democratization. Peace is a prerequisite to development. Democracy is essential if development is to succeed over the long term.

Real development of a State must be based on the participation of its population; that requires some form of democracy. To ensure such an achievement, democratization must not only take hold inside a State, but among States in the international community. Key factors are 1) international law, 2) human rights and 3) United Nations assistance to democratization.

The present decade is dedicated to international law. Virtually every aspect of what we call "the international community," is rooted in the great project of international law that began with Grotius over three centuries ago. It is a process to which distinguished lawyers of different parts of the world have contributed a great deal.

The importance of international law in dealing with settlement of conflict is obvious. Less obvious but equally important, international law is critical to development. A network of uniform commercial codes can speed commerce and link different cultures in common commitments. Economic transactions, from the smallest farmer to vast global corporations, insist on reliability. That requires rules that span borders, and mechanisms for the peaceful resolution of commercial disputes.

The cause of human rights has advanced considerably in the last two decades. The agreements signed by European nations at Helsinki in 1975 made it possible, for the first time in international law, to hold a State to a standard of universal conduct. No longer could regimes reject the outside world. No longer could they claim that the rights they denied were an "internal matter".

Human rights are principles of value in themselves. But they also make practical sense. Development cannot fully succeed where human rights are neglected. This is the age of information. And it is the age of people-centered development. People must be free to think, act and communicate not only as political but as economic beings. So human rights become a pillar of development.

Human rights. Equal rights. Government under law. Economic possibility. Freedom of thought and speech. Individual involvement and governmental accountability: all are the attributes of democratization.

Throughout most of this century and the last, democracy was regarded as something possessed by a few fortunate States and practiced within their borders. The international scene was defined by power politics. A balance of power provided an international system for the nations of the world; democracy among States was not even considered as a possibility.

The United Nations Charter offered a new vision. With its opening words "We the Peoples of the United Nations," democratization was built into the world organization. Even States whose internal politics were not democratic joined themselves in a representative parliament in which all States large and small were equal. The United Nations is taking on a wide array of new responsibilities to assist the progress of democratization within States.

In recent years the United Nations has ventured into an entirely new field: long-term, nation-wide monitoring of human rights. The first example was in El Salvador, in the context of the peace agreement which brought an end to the armed conflict in that country. A second is under way in Guatemala.

The UN sent missions to study the situation of human rights in Lithuania and Estonia. This was conceived as an effort of preventive diplomacy to defuse tensions between those nations and the Russian Federation.

In the Secretariat in New York during my tenure as Secretary General of the United Nations, I created a new office whose purpose, in essence, is to deal with electoral assistance requests by Member States as part of our efforts to promote democratization. In the short period since 1992, this office has handled dozens and dozens of requests from Asian States, Eastern European States, Latin America and Africa. All these requests are related to technical assistance, to the sending of observers and to electoral assistance. It should be borne in mind that until very recently, when it was decided to monitor the elections in Nicaragua in 1990, which opened the door to peace in that country, the United Nations regularly turned down all but technical assistance requests. We have since successfully monitored dozens of elections. But democracy within States can only be fully sustained over time if linked to increasing democratization among States and at all levels of the international system.

Among States, the United Nations is providing a framework for democratization. It is a forum where all voices can be heard. It provides a means of consensus-building. Preserving the moral authority of the United Nations requires the fullest participation and engagement of all States. This, in turn, calls for the involvement of all levels of international life: non-governmental organizations, academic institutions, parliamentarians, business and professional communities, the media and the public at large. It also means applying the principles of democratization within the United Nations itself. The time has come to fulfill the logic of the Charter and pursue not only democratization within States, but democratization throughout the international system.

These then are the three great tasks of the United Nations as set down by the Charter:

Without peace, there can be no development and there can be no democracy.

Without development, there can be no democracy and, without the basic elements of well-being, societies will disintegrate and enter into disputes.

Without democracy, no real development can occur. And without such development, peace cannot long be maintained.

Thus the three great priorities are interlocked.

At the heart of this interconnection will be the difficult question raised by timing among peace, development and democracy. In some cases, peace, development and democracy have been pursued and achieved simultaneously. Such was the case in El Salvador and Mozambique where the United Nations effort in support of democratization served as a link between conflict resolution, on the one hand and reconstruction and development on the other. In other cases, however, the joint pursuit of these 3 goals has proved more difficult at times, contributing to political instability, social disarray, and economic crisis.

Democratization requires as a precondition the achievement within a nation of a certain level of peace and a certain level of development. Both development and peace are essential yet the articulation between development and democracy is more complex.

Let us conclude then by trying to understand this complexity by formulating 4 basic rules:

1) Experience has shown that development cannot take place without democracy.

2) There is no one model of democratization or democracy suitable to all societies.

3) Each State must be free to decide for itself its priorities for the welfare of its people.
4) Democratization within States must also be supported by a process of democratization among States.

I want to express my gratitude once again to Professor Cahill and the Royal College of Surgeons in Ireland for the privilege of delivering this Distinguished International Health Lecture.

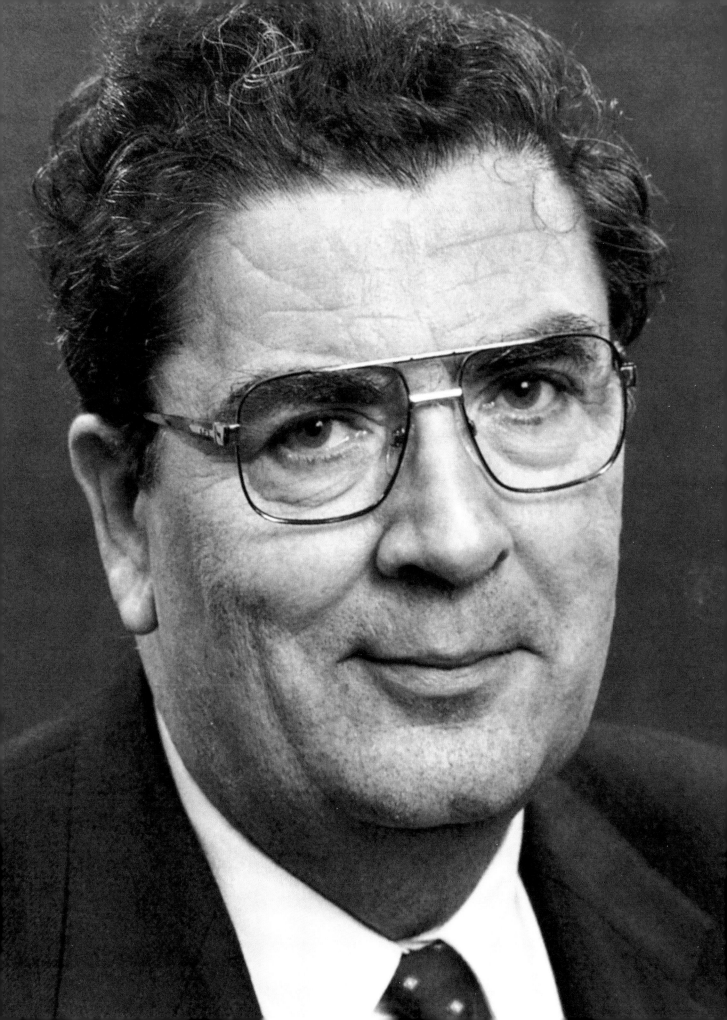

John Hume

His Distinguished International Lecture was delivered in the College on November 6, 1995.

John Hume was awarded the Nobel Peace Prize in 1998. His tireless, forty-year-plus, non-violent struggle in Northern Ireland has been praised around the world, and made him among the most admired persons in the island of Ireland. He had long served as Member of the European Parliament. He was the Founder and Leader of the Social Democratic Labour Party (SDLP) in Northern Ireland. His courageous, self-effacing negotiations with all parties to the conflicts in Northern Ireland is largely credited for the signing of the Good Friday Agreement in 1998, the foundation for the cessation of hostilities and the beginning of an evolving peace process.

Peace and the Healing Process
John Hume

Politics as a healing profession is the theme of my address this evening.

In one of the most famous pieces of political oratory – the Gettysburg Address – Abraham Lincoln spoke at the end of bloody civil war about binding the wounds of the nation. This is probably the most famous example of medical analogies being used to describe problems being suffered by, or processes being proffered to, the body politic.

It is not uncommon to hear people despair about the cancer of sectarianism or racism. References are made to paralysis, situations haemorrhaging, crippling effects, pain, hurt, trauma, fractures, mental scars and prognoses in many political commentaries, not only in situations where violence is, or has been, waging.

Over the years I have often talked of Ireland's need for a "healing process" and cautioned against notions of "instant cures." On numerous occasions I have found myself advising people to diagnose and treat causes of our political condition instead of scratching or picking at symptoms.

Medical or health analogies are particularly understandable in the context of a dysfunctional polity. They probably proliferate especially in circumstances where such political dysfunctionalism manifests itself in violence creating trauma which is all to real and literal.

The medical profession has to treat the consequences of such violence. In our own situation it has done so with distinction, dedication and determined co-operation spanning all levels and branches of the profession and associated professions.

From my perspective the political profession has to identify, isolate and treat the causes of such conflict. Unfortunately a comparable concerted effort involving all politicians to match the response to challenge by the clinicians has not yet been brought about—yet!

This can partly be explained by the fact that violence itself generates secondary political malignancies and complications. As Martin Luther King said, "Violence as a way of achieving justice is both impractical and immoral. It is impractical because it is a descending spiral ending in destruction for all. The old law of an eye for an eye leaves everybody blind. It is immoral because it seeks to humiliate the opponent rather than win his understanding, it seeks to annihilate rather than convert. Violence is immoral because it thrives on hatred rather than love. It destroys community and makes brotherhood impossible. It leaves society in monologue rather than dialogue."

Recognising that violence can only frustrate what we want to further and end up destroying what it starts out claiming to defend we must see if we can isolate violence itself. The effects of violence are preventing and undermining successful treatment of our underlying problem. Only by securing total relief from violence can we progress from monologue to the dialogue which is needed to treat our problem and help us towards the healing process.

Securing relief from the harrowing and debilitating secondary condition or symptoms does not constitute a cure. Nor does it lessen the need to go on to deal with the underlying problem. We need to be resolved rather than reluctant about moving on to the other phases or episodes of treatment and care without which we cannot have a healthy outcome. That is why I am concerned about the lack of movement, in this welcome absence of violence, by the British Government which is supposed to be a sponsor of the process at hand.

I can understand fears, misgivings and nervousness about the process ahead. It will be uncomfortable for all of us, but we have no alternative course to stability. People want cures but we do not like undergoing operations; just like people want to go to heaven but nobody wants to die. It is surprising what some people will tolerate in terms of toothache before submitting to a dentist.

I suppose we have a particular phobia about losing something. In our situation those in all traditions have an innate fear about having to give something up even if it is only vestigial. Anyone planning a successful intervention should be sensitive to such fears without being completely constrained by them. Feeding fears will not build confidence and comfort necessary for us to undergo and undertake the appropriate interventions and exercises.

As you can tell by now I am given to the idea that politics is concerned with healing the wounds of society, just as you heal the wounds of individuals. Given the attitudes of many people towards politics and its practitioners, this might seem an exaggerated or downright presumptuous claim. Nevertheless, I would argue strongly that healing is what politics should be about.

Of course, conflict and division is the foundation of politics, just as disease and injury is an essential prerequisite for the medical profession. If there were no divisions and difference of opinion in society, there would be no need for politics, just as there would be no need for doctors if there was no illness. But just as no doctor welcomes disease or injury for the sake of it, no politician should welcome conflict. To do otherwise is to betray the trust our fellow citizens put in us.

There are a number of similarities between medicine (in which as a layman I include surgery) and politics which I would like to consider for a few moments. There are also considerable differences which I will examine afterwards.

First, we have a common interest in healing. While you heal individuals, we as politicians have to deal with the defects of society. While you tackle disease and injury, we have to deal with the problems of poverty, unemployment, and in much of the world, violence. Of course, it would be naive to believe that there is no connection between the individual illnesses you treat and the social ills we as politicians have to address.

Second, I think we have a common awareness of the limitations of our knowledge and powers. Despite the great progress made over the years, there are still diseases which cannot be cured; there are still great social evils we have yet to overcome. Indeed, the great successes of the past are not irreversible. No advance is permanent. Each step forward has to be fought for again and again. It is not realistic to expect miracle cures. We cannot resolve immediately all the problems we face. But we can play a part in paving the way for eventual solutions.

That is why we have to take a long-term approach, playing our part in developments whose beneficiaries will be future generations. We have to do our best to make breakthroughs, to build on existing achievements and to prepare the future. We cannot necessarily offer the 'Promised Land' but we should be pointing in the right direction.

As far as the differences are concerned, the major one is the respectful gap between achievement and aspiration in our respective professions. While the medical profession has a solid record of achievement, politics and politicians often fail to live up to their aspirations. The outline above of the nature of politics obviously contains a degree of aspirational thinking on my own part rather than being simply a description of politics as it is today. That is not necessarily a criticism since politics is the realm *par excellence* of aspiration, and without it we would still be living in caves.

The problem occurs when politicians decide that their role is simply to articulate and reflect the divisions in society. In a divided society such as ours in Ireland, every public representative is, to a greater or larger extent, a reflection of the deep divisions that exist. That is inescapable; but one does not have to resign oneself to such a limited role, or even worse, make one's *raison d'être*. There is a challenge to extend ourselves to leadership rather than to content ourselves with spokespersonship alone.

Unlike doctors, we do not have to swear an oath to do no harm. It probably would not solve anything if we did, given that the divisions in our society mean that oaths are contentious in themselves. But I believe that the real purpose of politics, and the justification of political leadership, is to find ways of overcoming such divisions. Our moral duty is to find a way in which the people of this divided island can agree on how to share it and to begin the process of healing.

A further substantial difference between politics and medicine is the relative weight given to diagnosis. A doctor uses the symptoms to diagnose the illness; too many politicians use the symptoms to ignore the underlying political problems. The cycles of violence which have so disfigured our history perpetuated themselves because they were seen as the problem, not as a symptom of a general political failure to create adequate political institutions. In this divided island only institutions which will accommodate the different traditions on the island can guarantee a peaceful and democratic future. We need institutions which allow for the expression rather than the suppression of difference.

I have spent many years stressing the need for a serious diagnosis of the nature of the problem in Ireland, for which there was often much criticism. Indeed, I would argue without an adequate definition of the problem and some degree of consensus on the diagnosis, it is impossible to treat it. Without some minimum degree of agreement on the nature of the problem, we would be restricted to the political equivalent of using leeches. But I was, and remain, convinced that the progress made so far towards a peaceful island has been greatly facilitated by the gradual development of a minimal consensus on diagnosis, though quite naturally the prescriptions remain extremely diverse.

I would also like to point out one other major difference between politics and surgery. We operate without anaesthesia, even though some political leaders see themselves as amateur anaesthetists. It is not the job of public representatives to provide unjustified reassurance to their supporters. It is our job to tell our supporters that we have serious problems to overcome and that can only be done if we are all prepared to engage in a radical re-examination of our presuppositions and prejudices and inherited hatreds. We should refuse to even offer the prospect of pseudo-anaesthesia; it is our duty to inform and convince our fellow citizens of the need to take an active part in the creation of a new dispensation in our divided Ireland. This is perhaps the equivalent of the important role of Health Education and awareness programmes.

Bearing this in mind, I would like to emphasise a certain number of principles which have been important in the peace process so far, and indeed form the basis of the success so far achieved in silencing the guns. These principles will continue to underpin our strategy in the future.

First, we must address the problem of difference. There are three options in the face of difference: to pretend it does not exist; to combat such differences; or to accommodate them. We have seen the failure of the Stalinist attempt to pretend that difference either does not exist or is an irrelevance. We have all been sickened by the efforts of the warlords in ex-Yugoslavia to eradicate difference by killing and ethnic cleansing. In Ireland, the eradication of difference has been a regrettable part of our history. We have also suffered from the activities of those who thought that being Irish or British was a matter of life and death and who were prepared to make sure that it was. It seems to me, therefore, that the only rational, human and realistic course of action is to try to seek arrangements which will allow different traditions to live together while preserving their identities.

The only sensible way forward is to accept difference as inevitable and see it as a basic and a natural principle of human society. Indeed, with their advances in DNA analysis, we have the scientific proof that difference is universal. We must cherish the diversity of cultures which exist in Ireland, and seek to preserve them and the equilibrium between them.

In this respect, we can draw a great deal of inspiration from the existence of the European Union as living proof that a solution can be found. The European Union is the greatest-ever example of conflict resolution in human history. The fact is that countries which had spent centuries invading, occupying, expelling and massacring each other came together freely to put aside their past hatreds. They came together to work in their common interests and to ensure that war could no longer be a way to settling their differences. This in itself would have been remarkable but the fact that these countries will preserve their identities is even more encouraging.

It proves that it is possible to establish institutions which allow for common policies without submerging the variety of cultures and traditions which are real riches. The experience of the European Union therefore affords a good many lessons for those of us who still have to deal with the consequences of difference being perceived as a threat, both in Ireland and further afield. Without seeking to impose a particular political blueprint, I am convinced that there is much which can be adapted from the European Union for our eventual domestic use.

The second principle is that force, or the threat of force, is not a useful method of dealing with difference. Indeed, it often reinforces identities which might otherwise be only a minor part of a person's life. The use of force also generates more force, creating the vicious cycle of 'an eye for an eye.' The use of violence merely makes problems more intractable, as I have indicated earlier.

Third, differences can only be accommodated by dialogue and agreement. The basis for the cease-fires by both loyalists and republicans is the acceptance of this principle. Those organisations previously involved in violence now agree that only through negotiation can a suitable settlement be worked out. Neither side can force the other to accept the unacceptable. The peace has held because of the common commitment to agreement. It is time we moved on to serious talks on the content of an eventual political accord supported by all traditions in Ireland.

Fourth, we must be imaginative about political structures. No one should be scared of political change *per se*; though clearly change must be brought about by agreement. Bur change is as fundamental to human society as diversity. Without it, stagnation is inevitable. Stagnation itself is a cause of conflict just as its biological equivalent causes degeneracy and disease.

It is also necessary to ensure that political institutions are adapted to the needs of citizens rather than mould the citizen to suit the purposes of the institutions. In a divided society it is therefore vital that the institutions reflect the needs and aspirations of all sections of society. Creating institutions which can command the consent of all citizens of whatever identity is not a simple task, but there is no doubt that it can be done. In many countries, there are complex political arrangements which are not that easy to understand as an outsider, but which command the support of the overwhelming majority of their citizens.

We should not be afraid of complexity and diversity in our political systems. Complexity and diversity are increasingly recognised by scientists as the crucial organising factors in the natural world. Why shouldn't it be the same in the social and political world, if anything, society and the political system should be even more complex than the natural world? We should not be worried about creating complex political structures if their purpose and effect is to create an inclusive system capable of securing the allegiance of all citizens of all traditions. What we should denounce are systems, simple or complex, which serve to exclude citizens of any or all traditions from the decision-making process.

Where does this leave us? The most urgent requirement now is to overcome the obstacles to comprehensive all-party negotiations. Though we have succeeded in putting a stop to violence, we have yet to make the peace.

There is a long way to got before a political settlement can be concluded to which all sections of our divided people can give their allegiance. Such a settlement will be necessary if our people are to look forward to a future where all our energies are devoted to overcoming the massive political, economic and social challenges facing our society. We have to ensure that the conflict which has so disfigured our society becomes and remains a distant and tragic memory.

To achieve this goal will take a great deal of effort. It will require all of us to examine our traditional assumptions and preconceptions. It will take a lot of hard thinking and tough talking. It will require serious negotiations in which all relevant parties to the conflict engage in the overriding task of finding new political arrangements which will reflect the interests and aspirations of all traditions in Ireland.

The keys to the eventual political understanding for which all our people are crying out can, therefore, be easily identified: the need for a speedy beginning to all-inclusive negotiations: and the recognition that an acceptable political system can only be created by agreement. There is no place for any form of duress, physical or moral, in the creation of new genuinely democratic institutions. Nor is there any room for the type of thinking which is dominated by notions of victory and defeat. The successful creation of an Ireland at peace and striving for prosperity can only be a victory for all traditions, just as violence, conflict, and the absence of peace are a defeat for us all.

It is also clear that the need for agreement on the future of Northern Ireland is generally accepted by all parties and by the Irish and British governments. The Downing Street Declaration made this clear, as have subsequent comments by the various parties and the two governments. The task is not for the divided peoples of Ireland to work out an agreement on the ways in which we can share our island. Both governments have made it clear that they accept the right of our people to define their own future political institutions and that their wishes will not be overridden by either state. The British government, for instance, has made it clear that it has no selfish or strategic motive to hold on to Northern Ireland against the will of its people. It is up to us, the people of Ireland, North and South, unionist and nationalist, to map out an agreement.

Having said that, it is important that the opportunity to create political agreement in Ireland for the first time is seized as rapidly as possible. We therefore believe that all-inclusive talks should take place at the earliest possible date. We do not think it is helpful to impose pre-conditions on such talks, since the whole purpose of negotiating is to surmount the difficulties which the pre-conditions undoubtedly reflect. We prefer to address the underlying conditions from which pre-conditions emerge, concentrating on the problem rather than the symptoms.

The crucial task is to take the gun out of Irish politics once and for all. The only way we can do that is to tackle the problems of division, mistrust, and hatred which led people to resort to violence in the first place.

Since the cessations of violence, the major preliminary question has been answered. Groups formerly committed to the use of force have made it clear that they are prepared to enter into negotiations on the understanding that they are determined to use exclusively peaceful and political methods to pursue their objectives. That is the major touchstone for all-inclusive negotiations. We believe that no serious government or political force in these islands could fail to seize this unprecedented opportunity.

While we are convinced that all-inclusive negotiations are the only possible route to peace, we do not underestimate the difficulties involved in bringing about a successful conclusion. Clearly, the parties involved have considerable difference of opinion which will not be changed overnight. Our history of violence and conflict has left many wounds which will not easily heal. The extent of poverty and deprivation has alienated many people of all traditions from the political process. We do not have a culture of negotiation and agreement.

But we are totally convinced that an eventual political

agreement is feasible and can be brought to fruition. Three reasons can be cited: the underlying common interests of our citizens: international support for the peace process: and the emergence of political agreements in other divided societies throughout the world.

Despite our political differences, our traditions have a common interest in peace and in economic prosperity. There is a vast area of economic and social policy where our divided peoples are united and where we can work together without compromising on deeply and sincerely held convictions. We can spill our sweat and not our blood and so build the necessary trust to heal our deeper divisions. As a peripheral region of the European Union, we have a common interest in adopting a united approach to our European partners, just as we have such a common interest in our relations with the rest of the world. We have a common interest in developing our economic position within the global economy and in establishing fair patterns of trade in international markets. The more we get used to pursuing our common interests, the more we can address our political divisions.

Second, the support and goodwill of our friends in the European Union, the US and the Commonwealth is an asset of enormous value. The interest shown in the peace process in the outside world is very helpful in building confidence among our peoples and in combating the tendency to think in narrow and self-defeating terms. Seeing how diverse peoples throughout the world have ordered their affairs is a useful corrective against an excessively Anglo- or Hiberno-centric view of the world.

Finally, the emergence of peace processes in divided societies in other parts of the world is a massive boost for confidence in the possibility of negotiated agreements. I am thinking for instance of South Africa where the work of Nelson Mandela and F. W. de Kierk has produced an agreement far more successful than anyone thought possible even two years ago. We will have to find our own way, just as South Africa did. The real lesson we take is that, given sufficient determination and imagination, political structures which respect diversity and difference and which reconcile former enemies, are possible and indeed the only path to peace.

Just as with many medical interventions and treatments we cannot guarantee that there is absolutely no risk. But without taking a course with its element of possible risk there may be no hope of recovery.

We are gathered here on the day of Yitzhak Rabin's funeral. He grew from being a brave soldier to being a brave statesman. He latterly embraced in the Middle East the profound value of what Olof Palme tried to tell the Cold War world – we can only truly be secure with each other, not against each other. With Shimon Peres, Yasser Arafat and others he took risks for peace, just as he took personal risks in war. Indeed a public exhortation of the need to take risks for peace were among his last words at the peace rally where he was assassinated.

As we think of this man who has helped to build peace in the 'Promised Land' and offer our hope and help for peace in that region, we can usefully reflect on some words from another assassinated leader. One who said on the eve of his death, "…I have seen the promised land. I may not get there with you. But I want you to know that we as a people will get to the promised land."

On an earlier occasion Martin Luther King offered counsel which is valuable for the motivation and morale of clinicians and politicians alike and relevant to frustrations now being experienced – "We must accept finite disappointment, but we must never lose infinite hope."

He also challenged all of us to reach beyond the confines of our given orthodoxies or our own local and subjective perspectives and to embrace mutual acceptance and human solidarity. He offered a most meaningful interpretation for health and wealth in this world and at the same time tried to rally us above notions of narrow nationalism. With words that are a most appropriate reference for an international health lecture Martin Luther King said:

"As long as there is poverty in the world I can never be rich even if I have a billion dollars. As long as diseases are rampant and millions of people in this world cannot expect to live more than twenty-eight or thirty years, I can never be totally healthy even if I just got a good check-up at Mayo Clinic. I can never be what I ought to be until you are what you ought to be. This is the way our world is made. No individual or nation can stand out boasting of being independent. We are interdependent."

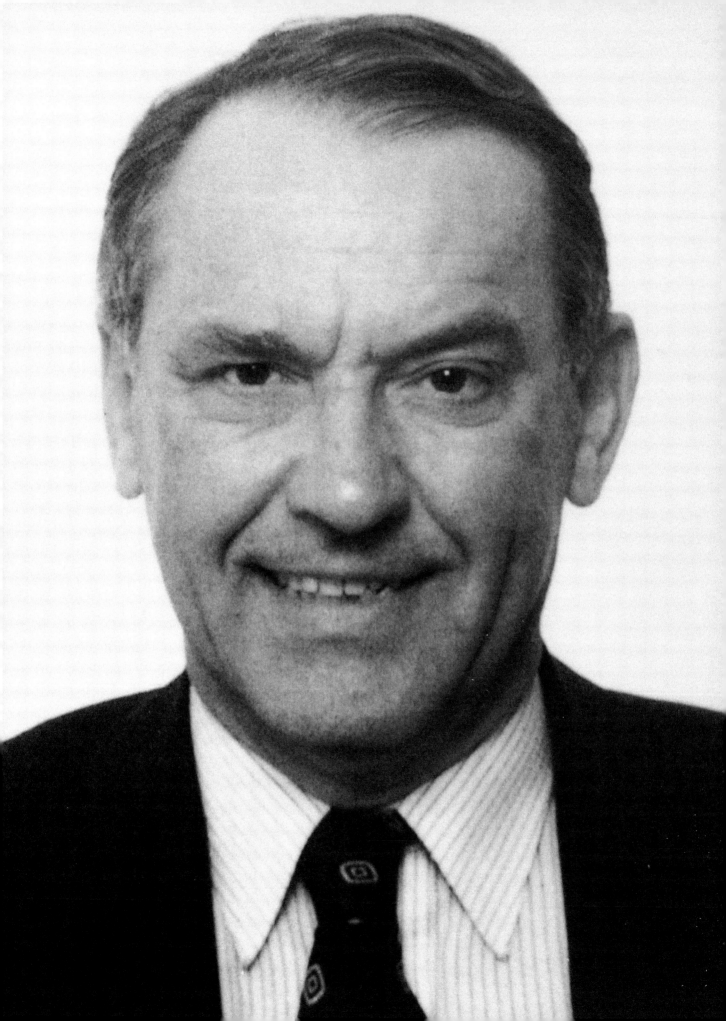

Jan Eliasson

*His Distinguished International Lecture was delivered
in the College on November 7, 1994.*

Jan Eliasson is currently Deputy Secretary-
General of the United Nations. He was President
of the 60th Session of the U.N. General
Assembly, while contemporaneously serving as
the Foreign Minister of Sweden. Throughout
his distinguished diplomatic career, he has
been deeply involved in fostering humanitarian
efforts in the search for peace. He was the first
UN Under-Secretary-General for Humanitarian
Affairs. He served as Personal Representative of
the UN Secretary-General during the Iran-Iraq
conflict and in the Darfur negotiations. He has
been a Visiting Professor at Upsala University,
among others, in international affairs. He was a
Director of the CIHC. He has received numerous
awards and honorary degrees from governments
and universities around the world.

A World in Turmoil: the Imperative of Prevention
Jan Eliasson

I thank you very much, Kevin, for your very generous and very personal introduction. We have done a lot of work together, Professor Cahill and I. We are united in that fraternity of people committed to the humanitarian cause. I applaud Kevin Cahill, not only as President of the Center for International Humanitarian Cooperation or as Professor at this distinguished College, but as the Kevin Cahill who stood up for the humanitarian needs and work that should be done in Somalia, and also the Kevin Cahill who has just authored a book, *Clearing the Fields: Solutions to the Global Landmine Crisis,* an extremely important contribution regarding a massive problem that we have to deal with very soon and in a very practical way.

On a lighter note I am glad though that you did not introduce me as when I delivered a speech in New York just eight months ago. There the woman seemed to read my entire Curriculum Vitae and then she ended by saying "and may I introduce to you the man responsible for all disasters in the world." So thank you for avoiding that approach.

I am also very glad to be in Ireland. Today I have had very interesting talks in the Foreign Ministry about the European Union. The Swedish people must decide whether they shall vote in favour or against joining the European Union on Sunday of this week. It is very important for our nation, and it was very important for me, to have the discussions today and to identify how much Ireland and Sweden are indeed like minded. You know the wonderful quote from Shakespeare's *"Romeo and Juliet"* when he reminded us, about the 1580's or

'90's, that "there is a world outside Verona."

Ireland and Sweden in common, know that there is a world outside Verona, and that we have to deal with that reality, and that we cannot build our security in isolation, in an island of prosperity. Rather we must build it on global responsibility and global commitment. That is why I hope the Swedish people will take the wise decision and join Ireland in building a new European architecture as well as contribute to the global architecture of security at the end of the Cold War.

I also want to note that during my work in the international humanitarian field I met so many Irish people in very concrete situations; I want you to know how much I appreciated your Irish soldiers in Lebanon (who paid a very heavy price by the way), and the Irish nurses in Somalia. I still see in front of me the brave nurses who did fantastic work in Baidoa and where again a great personal price had to be paid for that courageous work I also enjoyed the meeting with your President, Mrs. Robinson, when she visited the Secretary General in New York. I found an unusual commitment at the highest level from your Government and your society. So, we have a lot to do outside Verona.

Now the title of my presentation is "A World in Turmoil: The Imperative of Prevention." It will be one descriptive part and one prescripted part; the turmoil is the analytical descriptive side, the prevention is the prescripted side. I thought that it would be a fitting theme, on this occasion of meeting so many physicians and surgeons, to emphasize prevention, to show how much there is in common between the professions of medicine and those of diplomacy and international politics. What I will propose as my most important message is that we have to move the focus from dealing with symptoms to dealing with primary causes. We have to learn how to translate early warning into early action. If I may use medical language, with all due respect for the heart surgeons, I know from personal experience with heart surgeons that they are frantically looking for more action in the preventive side so that the patients will not come, in extremis, to them in the great numbers that they are doing today. Surgeons are now emphasizing, for instance, the important role of dieticians who can tell you what to eat and what not to eat if you are to avoid the traumatic moment of a heart operation, or at least it can be avoided as long as possible or made less frequent than today.

If you translate that approach to the political arena you will see what I mean; I will start with the turmoil. In this first part I would like to identify two factors that I think are now creating the conditions for international co-operation and are, in fact, setting the stage for the type of work that can be done, and also, perhaps, setting some restrictions on what can be done. I will stress two factors; one is the end of the Cold War, and the second is the great increase in internal crises. To put it very simply, there is an explosion of civil wars around the world, often with religious and ethnic elements.

When the Cold War ended around 1989, when the wall tumbled down in Europe, I think we recognised the enormous potential in the end of that very absurd period of modern history. I think we were all nurturing a hope that now was the time to move from merely looking at nations as pawns in a geopolitical strategic chess game. Rather we could now see nations as societies with human beings who have the right of political freedom, economic and social justice. In other words we could truly put the human being in the centre, rather than focus on nations and states as cold parts of a puzzle.

Translating this in the United Nations, where I spent six years very recently, has meant, at the end of the Cold War, that the veto of the Security Council is more or less gone. The veto has been used only once in the last four years in the Security Council on a simple matter concerning the financing of the operations in Cyprus. You may recall how in the '50's, '60's, '70's and early '80's the debilitating United Nations veto stopped almost any significant action. There was the Soviet veto in the '50's, and even worse vetoes in the '60's, '70's and '80's on South Africa and the Middle East. You may not recall that the Vietnam War, which was such a big issue for my generation, and for many of yours, was never even debated in the Security Council. You may recall that famous moment when Adlai Stevenson pointed at the Russian Soviet missiles behind him at the Security Council; but that famous debate was not followed by a resolution. You may recall that Afghanistan, at the beginning of that conflict, never even came up for discussion. Why? Because everybody knew that a veto would stop any meaningful action.

So now today's Vietnam, today's Afghanistan, come up in the Security Council and are being discussed, as with Bosnia or Somalia. So today the United Nations gets all the difficult conflicts. The Security Council is now an effective body, sometimes to the degree that the UN is criticised more for doing too much, as in Somalia, than for doing too little, as sometimes has been the case in Yugoslavia.

The end of the Cold War has also meant that there is less competition among the major powers for influence and favours in the developing countries. This, to some extent, is positive. I think mainly it is positive that the developing nations are being left alone. But the negative side of it is also that resources are not flowing to the developing world to the extent that they were in the past, because that super-power political competition is gone. All in all, however, I think we all must agree that the end of the Cold War is good news and that it is, of course, to be welcomed.

Now I come to my second aspect of the major change in modern times, and that is the explosion of civil wars, caused by a release of pent-up internal forces. It is as though the wet blanket of the Cold War has been lifted away and you have now factors which for too long were suppressed, exploding in our face. Even the world map is changing, because the Cold War kept nations under control and there was a lack of democracy and participation in many countries. Now with the Cold War disappearing, and the growth of democracy and participatory processes, internal forces take over and shape developments.

This course has led to a tendency towards fragmentation, a tendency to micro nationalism. Nations are being divided along ethnic and religious lines. This is something I basically react against because it gives a message that we cannot live together if we belong to different ethnic and religious groups. This is not what we should want to teach our children

In fact, there is a positive tendency in these changes for the result is, of course, to emphasize the rights of minorities, human rights and to identity different forms for oppressed minorities. In political terms, we must now ask ourselves whether solidarity ends at a national border or whether solidarity ends with a human being in need.

The Pol Pot genocide of the seventies was an absolutely unbelievable event which really did not cause the kind of reaction that you today see in the Somalia and Rwanda situations. I do not think that we have done enough for either Somalia or Rwanda, but the question is no longer even asked whether the international community has a responsibility inside a country if there is a widespread humanitarian crisis.

The resolution that created the United Nations Department of Humanitarian Affairs, that I was the first one to head, included two very important commitments from governments. One was an acceptance that every government has a responsibility for the well-being of its own population. A very simple but also very powerful statement. Secondly, it was agreed that every government has the responsibility to provide access to people in need in humanitarian crisis.

With those two tools in my hands I could negotiate, in war torn Sudan, the opening of humanitarian corridors from Kenya into Southern Sudan. I know by that action that we saved many thousands of lives. It was a sort of infringement on national sovereignty but with the consent and agreement of the government in question. By the fact that they have accepted the principle of access, and the principle of responsibility for their own population, they actually had opened the border. Solidarity did not automatically stop at the border. This is very new.

We still have an organisation, the United Nations, which is based on sovereignty, on the UN Charter Article 27 of not interfering in internal affairs but we also have an organisation which now, more and more, is putting, and mind you should put, human beings in the centre. We must try to strike a proper balance between sovereignty and solidarity. This is the philosophical framework in which the United Nations is now working. It is both a dilemma and, in my view, a great challenge.

What does this mean for the United Nations, these changes, the end of the Cold War and the explosion of internal crises? I think the UN role is changed in three regards:

1) The UN role has become more active, getting inside national borders, not only monitoring cease-fires at the military border.

2) It has also become more comprehensive. The role is not only military; the role today includes political reconciliation, humanitarian work, development, rehabilitation, reconstruction, and dealing with the health clinics.

3) As a result of these said changes United Nations personnel are more exposed, and I mean both physically and politically. I saw that with my own eyes, out in so many areas of the world, losing people to an extent that we never did before, not only because we are out where the conflicts are but also, politically, the United Nations is sticking its neck out. We are becoming more controversial because we are inside nations sometimes taking a side in an internal situation.

Those three are very major changes. It means that peace keeping, the classical notion of peace keeping which you, the Irish, and we, the Swedish, know so well, is also changing character. Peace-keeping is not only a military exercise now. Peace-keeping includes political reconciliation and humanitarian action. I spent considerable time in Somalia and I saw with my own eyes how much could be done, and how much was not done, in the humanitarian arena. I know the effect that a good humanitarian programme could have on the need for a military component.

At one stage in the middle of 1993, for every dollar that we had for the humanitarian programme in Somalia we had to pay ten dollars for military protection. My programme was one hundred and sixty five million dollars a year in 1993. The programme for the military operation, with over thirty thousand men, cost 1.5 billion dollars and yet the primary objective of the whole exercise was to relieve the humanitarian crisis. I made that case publicly and said that I found this imbalance rather dangerous.

In fact, what we did not do in the humanitarian sector could have contributed to less need for military security. If we were to have taken away the mines, 1.5 million in Northern Somalia alone, we would have enhanced security. If we had built health clinics, mended the roads, built bridges, brought children to school; if we had given jobs to the young men who were brandishing their weapons at you, we would have made a major contribution to security. In other words humanitarian work, development work, rehabilitation work is an investment in security, and we shall see a growing dynamic interdependence between the military component, the political component and the humanitarian component. They belong together and create one entity. That is the type of peace keeping that I think is now necessary.

Now that brings me to the prescripted part. You will notice that I have already painted the prescripted section on the case of Somalia. We have to ask ourselves again – if this is the world we live in, at both the end of the Cold War, and with an explosion of civil wars around the globe – what can we then do? Generally, and almost philosophically, I think we now are facing a period in which the United Nations is almost overcharged and overworked. I think many of you, when you open the newspaper or watch television at night, ask yourself, what's next? This new country I have never even heard about is going to explode? This may lead to a sense of powerlessness. I think it is very important, therefore, to try to divide the problems into manageable parts. As Prime Minister Palme always said to me when I came and gave him a list of ten crises: "one hell at a time, please."

I think, therefore, it is important to try to sort out what can be done in each individual crisis. If you look at a specific crisis, and list the expectations on the United Nations, I think it is obvious that there are three things that can be done.

I will deal primarily with prevention. But there are the other things, of course, that one must do since the UN is getting all these challenges.

The UN must have the resources to do the job, financially and materially, in personnel and lorries. That is the first answer. Of course, they must also have the mandate to do the job. The second answer is that, perhaps, the United Nations should not do everything alone.

If we always say this is the fault of the United Nations, the UN is not doing this, they are not doing that, then we promote a dangerous "we, they, syndrome." The UN is us. But if we do not give the UN the resources to do the job we should perhaps consider a division of labour where regional organisations as well as the UN are carrying the responsibility. My negotiations recently on Nagorno-Karabach, was done for the OSEC, the Security and Co-operation Organization of Europe, not the UN. The UN Charter provides for regional co-operation as part of the job. Maybe also non-governmental organisations can do more. I was, as I said earlier, extremely helped by the NGO's in Somalia and Sudan. They gave early warning to conflicts and were extremely helpful. This leads to my main point.

After six years at the UN, and sometimes almost despairing experiences of seeing suffering around the world, I am convinced that it is in the field of prevention where we have to do the main work right now. I felt, being the First Under-Secretary for Humanitarian Affairs, responsible for disasters in the world, that we were working like firemen, night-shift and day-shift. And I was sometimes very angered that we were reacting only when the fire was visible. We talked about the CNN factor, but it was often only when CNN covered the crisis that we finally got attention to a problem. I could not morally and ethically accept that the chance of the survival of a child depends on uncovering that child's misery, yet that was the case. I said to myself: what can we do to move attention from the fire to perfecting techniques for identifying the arsonist when he puts the match to the house or, even better, identify the potential arsonist?

You can, of course, translate these questions into a lot of areas, political, diplomatic, social, economic, humanitarian and you will see what I mean. I think one of the most civilised moves that we can do, especially in countries like Ireland and Sweden, and among the many of you who are working with medical and humanitarian problems, is to see that we move our attention to the early stages of disasters. If we can do that we will, I think, foster and make an historic change, the best contribution to the post Cold War analysis.

My generation was not too good about making such innovations. I look at many of the young people here and ask that you please make this your priority – to move the attention from the fire to the identification of potential arsonist. Not only would we avoid a lot of suffering, if that is not enough, which I know it is for the people in this room, but also we would save a lot of money. There is an explosion in peace keeping and in humanitarian crises operations. We now pay four times more for peace keeping than we did five years ago. In the last four years alone the peace-keeping operations cost the same amount as for the whole history of the United Nations up until now.

We must not only deal with symptoms but focus on root causes. I thought about this when I was working with the South African drought. I do not know how many of you know that in 1992 Southern Africa went through its most serious drought in the history of recorded Africa. Eleven countries were threatened by famine; eighty million people were endangered. When I opened our Embassy in Zimbabwe, someone noted that the reservoir had only eight per cent of water left.

We made an international appeal and received seven hundred million dollars for eleven countries. It was distributed with a minimum, if any, corruption because everyone knew it involved a question of survival. The South Africans opened their ports; all the African ambassadors in New York agreed that this was indeed an exceptional case. We co-operated with the regional organisation, Southern Africa Development Community, and it worked. In order not to sound like I am bragging, I should record that we were saved by a little bit of rain in some areas and by positive developments in Angola and Mozambique at the time. But the operation worked. Now how many of you ever heard about this? I suppose very few. In other words prevention is not rewarded. Prevention is not seen. Please give me the mechanisms that make prevention noted. Where is the Nobel Peace Prize for prevention? The type of public attention that should be given to prevention is simply not there.

Prevention cannot be something one just speaks about. You must translate it into a concrete programme of action in the diplomatic and political field. If you have the first signal of a crisis, my proposition is that there are a number of things which start with early warning. In order not to be too general on this topic, I will give one specific example of what can be done through preventive diplomacy. Early warning may be the first signal from a young NGO in Southern Somalia that something is wrong, that there is a risk that this single pocket of misery that can lead to a hundred thousand people dying. He or she may send this information to CONCERN or CARE or Save the Children Organisation. The NGO then calls me as Under-Secretary General and I am responsible for action. We do not currently have a system that is well enough developed yet. We must learn to make use of the field information system and then translate early warning to early action. The first sign of a crisis must be taken seriously. We cannot disregard that first sign. The earlier we start the easier it is to solve a crisis and the less the costs are.

Let us now look at the United Nations Secretary General's role. The Secretary General can send fact finding missions; this may sound like a very bureaucratic thing. But imagine, for example, how helpful a fact finding mission can be by highlighting problems with a short visit to an area in Southern Sudan. Even private organizations can make significant contributions by using the fact finding mission technique. Jimmy Carter's Centre is one such organisation which has played an important role in sending fact finding missions to troubled spots from Haiti to Yugoslavia.

Then consider the potential in the UN Charter. The UN Charter contains a Chapter Six. It has a wonderful heading – Specific Peaceful Settlement of Disputes. Now in this chapter there is a specific list of what can be done. It is a very impressive list of things but ask yourself how often is this used? Negotiation, enquiry, mediation, conciliation, arbitration, judicial settlement, regional agents arrangements and other peaceful means of their own choice. This is what the opposing parties can use to find peaceful solutions.

Then we come to something we call in the UN, half jokingly, half seriously, "Chapter six and a half," which includes peace keeping operations to encourage peaceful settlements and action against certain international peace and security. Those operations, as I said earlier, should now be much more sophisticated, should contain both military, if this is necessary, political and humanitarian components to become truly effective as a step before force is used.

When you enter Chapter Seven of the UN Charter, you can actually use force. But Chapter Seven is not immediately an invitation to military force; Chapter Seven contains a section about sanctions. I am the first one to admit, as a person responsible for humanitarian affairs, that sanctions can indeed be a very blunt instrument because the people who are vulnerable can pay a very heavy price for sanctions. I have seen it with my own eyes in Iraq, Haiti and Yugoslavia, but it is, nonetheless, an instrument that can be used for peaceful change. If that instrument is made more precise, and is done in such a way that it hurts those who are really in power, like for instance freezing assets of rulers, it can be helpful. There is also another use of force and that is the threat of the use of force.

Well if you look at this whole range from early warning to fact finding missions, to Chapter six peaceful solutions, to Chapter six and a half sophisticated comprehensive peace keeping operations and on to sanctions and the threat of the use of force, it is a very impressive list of things, in my view, that can be done. I am trying to be very specific in my contention that prevention is not just a slogan. It is a list of things that we can do and which, in my view, are rarely done sufficiently. Now since I am a specialist in negotiation and diplomacy and politics then this is my diplomatic list. But one can translate this list, of course, to a similar approach on social, environmental warning signals, humanitarian warning signals, economic warning signals. Often one can see the risks of conflicts coming from the social and economic situation. I have stressed the diplomatic version since this is the area in which I specialise.

I would like to discuss another measure in this last topic, the threat to use force. Should that option be left? I must say that the United Nations would probably not be a relevant actor in the world if one did not have that possibility of reacting with force when no other means has worked. In the end there must be a last resort; for instance in facing Saddam Hussain's aggression to Kuwait. There has to be a time when it is clear that one will not reward aggression. Despite all I have said about prevention, of course, we must recognize that if all these measures fail there has to be a credible last alternative. I would say, however, that peace enforcement is not very effective today; once we come into peace enforcement situations when military force is used, and when the United Nations is tested, like in the case of Somalia, it turns out that the multi-lateral varnish can be rather thin.

When the United States lost eighteen men on the 3rd October, 1993, the US Congress and the US public opinion asked that the US leave Somalia immediately; five other countries quickly came to the same conclusion. It is not easy to have countries accept sacrifices in such situations, to the extent that their young men are dying in great numbers. I suppose this is the reason why we have not seen more resolve in Bosnia. It also shows in the last resort that it is probably preferable that there be a form of coalitions rather than a purely UN led operation.

In todays political climate, if the UN is to be effective, we should remember that the UN is basically a moral and ethical force. The first line of defence, not only for small and medium size countries, but for all people who are now exposed to violence in the world, is respect for international law, humanitarian law, and for human rights. The tasks of the United Nations, and of the entire international community was best formulated by the Brazilian delegation several years ago. They said the United Nations has three tasks – peace, development and a life in dignity for all. Peace and development are I think rather well known tasks for the United Nations but what is interesting is the formulation of a mandate for the international community to also work for a life in dignity for all.

All this means is that we now have a serious chance to put human beings in the centre, and to finally let the old Cold War rhetoric move aside. We enter a stage in history where we have respect for international law but also, and this is my main point, an appreciation of the imperative for prevention. If we can translate this message on prevention into a concrete programme of action we would make the most important contribution to a new kind of international co-operation that we must develop at this momentous stage in the story of mankind.

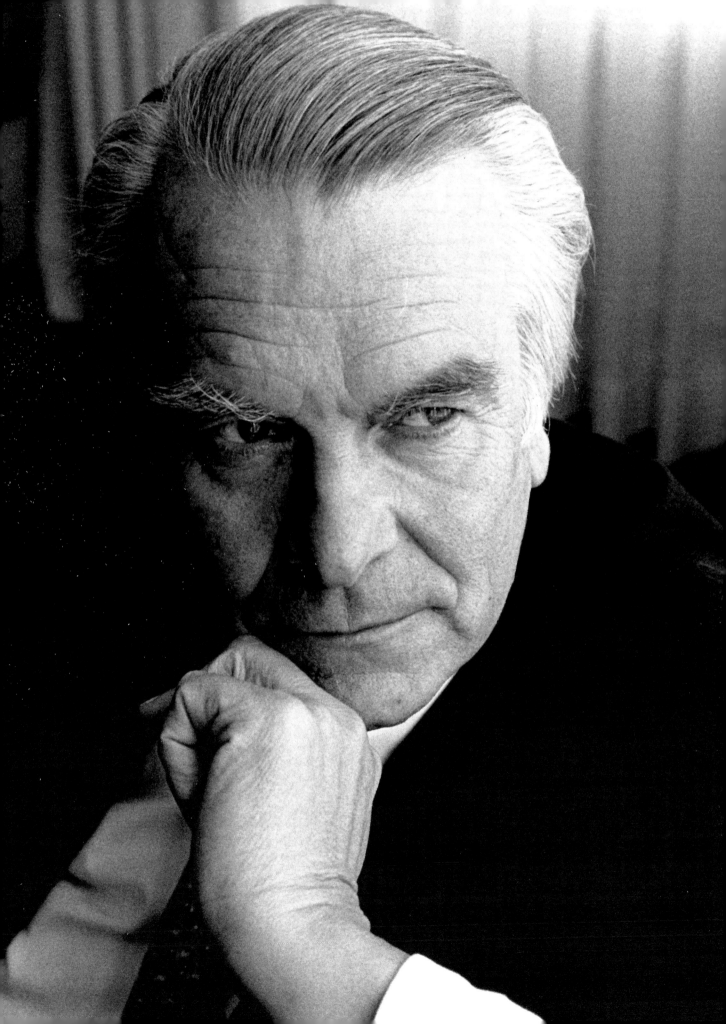

Lord David Owen

His Distinguished International Lecture was delivered in the College on November 8, 1993.

The Right Honorable the Lord Owen, CH, was a Member of the British Parliament for twenty-six years. He had graduated medical school at Cambridge University, and begun a promising career in neurology at St. Thomas's Hospital in London, when he entered political life. He subsequently served as Navy Minister, Health Minister, and Foreign Secretary of the United Kingdom. He was a Founder and Leader of the Social Democratic Party, the Chancellor of the University of Liverpool, the EU Co-Chairman of the International Conference on the Former Yugoslavia and the Chairman of Humanitas. He is a Director, and Secretary, of the CIHC. For those fortunate to know this multifaceted man well, his humanity and sensitivity may be best captured in his *Seven Ages of Man: Poetry for a Lifetime*, an anthology that links very clearly the diverse strands in this Lecture Series on Medicine, Art, and Foreign Policy.

Preventive Diplomacy:
The Therapeutics of Mediation
Lord David Owen

The Greek physician Herophilus observed some 2,000 years ago that illness "renders science null, art inglorious, strength effortless, wealth useless, and eloquence powerless." Conflict does much the same to the body politic. Conflict is cancerous in the way it erodes democracy and trust, brutalises behaviour and destroys civilised values and constraints. Preventing is very different from curing illness and preventive health has acquired over the centuries particular disciplines and skills. Preventing conflict also requires different skills from resolving conflict even though they cannot always be separated out. Yet diplomats, unlike physicians, have not fully developed a preventive ethos and a disciplined method of working.

The second half of the 19th century and the first half of the 20th Century has seen in the developed world a dramatic fall in mortality rates mainly attributable to the prevention of deaths from infectious diseases. Preventive public health measures to provide clean water supplies and improved housing have made, though it is not often recognised, a far more dramatic impact than clinical treatment. Prevention continues to do so through immunisation programmes. The WHO smallpox eradication campaign was a striking success and hopefully polio will soon follow. Yet tuberculosis is returning. Drug therapy, particularly antibiotics, has played their part, as have modern surgerical techniques and chemotherapy. There has also developed a counter-movement to ill judged medical interventions seen in the growth of life-style adjustments, homeopathic medicines and a greater readiness to rely on the body's own defence mechanisms.

Realistic doctors are only too well aware of the inadequacies of their skills when confronting much illness. It is a salutary fact that as the population lives longer the vast bulk of modern illness is not cured but alleviated by the doctor's skills. The majority of doctors', nurses' and therapists' time is spent in helping patients to accommodate themselves to the facts of their illness. The largest element in all illness in modern society is the ageing process itself – a largely irreversible process. Health services and the doctors are cast in the role of the providers of good health, yet, at best, for the bulk of illness all they can do is watch as the body wears itself out. The dramatic cure is the exception rather than the rule.

Much the same limitation affects politicians dealing with conflict within a nation or internationally. Violence is part of daily living; we can deplore its existence but we are not likely to be able to root it out from our diverse societies. The Cold War avoided a set battle between NATO and the Warsaw Pact – but there were surrogate battles between the US and the Soviet Union and many other conflicts which resulted in a hideous loss of life. Despite the UN providing a framework for international order and world peace its first 50 years was sadly characterised by multiple wars. The possibility of the UN intervening in a conflict within a nation-state was virtually excluded after the Korean war; but interventions had a short lived vogue from 1990-92. Yet the disappointing results mean that even the principle of such interventions is now having to be critically reassessed. It has also become clear that we do not know enough about the multifaceted impact of economic and trade sanctions as well as differing forms of military intervention. The doctor and the politician are not as different as perhaps both, and in particular the doctor, would like to think. Each is essentially involved in the practice of natural science. The physicist and engineer deal in absolutes. The clinician and the politician can only use science as an aid; and they are both intimately involved in human behaviour. Inevitably in their decision-making they fuse, not only scientific and statistical evidence, but also important elements of the behavioural sciences. Both have to relate their decisions to, and identify with a multiplicity of human variables. The doctor is primarily involved with, the individual; the national politician inevitably predominantly with groups of individuals, the statesman with groupings of nations. The skill of the good politician and the skill of the good clinician comes not just from their ability to observe life, to understand and feel a concern for their fellow men and women, but also from knowing when to intervene and when to leave alone. The greatest mistakes in politics and medicine often derive from an inability to comprehend and anticipate the underlying trends and developments affecting individuals. I have adapted an old prayer of Sir Robert Hutchinson, a 19th Century physician at the London Hospital, into a "Politician's Prayer":

"From inability to let well alone, from too much zeal for the new and contempt for what is old, from putting knowledge before wisdom, science before art and cleverness before commonsense, from treating individuals as statistics and for making change in the body politic more grievous than the endurance of the same, good Lord deliver us".

Just as the wise clinician understands that the body has an ability to heal itself so the wise politician knows that the body politic too has its own correcting mechanisms. If one intervenes to correct one factor, an imbalance will often appear somewhere else. The good clinician can never diagnose or treat any symptom in isolation: the whole man embraces his environment just as much as his ailment. In politics exactly the same factors have to be reckoned with, for an interventionist style of politics, is an exposed one and any action will be clearly related to the change it may introduce – positive or adverse. Inaction and immobility in politics, as in medicine, can exaggerate or perpetuate tendencies that already exist so that they become damaging. Intervention, on the other hand, is capable of wreaking far more havoc than inaction. The interventionist politician, like the interventionist clinician, therefore, has a duty to commission research and pay respect to the results of any such research. An intervention which is not based on much factual evidence as is available is simply irresponsible.

Yet just as doctors and politicians can only work on the margin of human behaviour and existence, society still thinks they have far greater power than in reality they possess. "Do something!" remains a common cry. However, the frustration the doctor feels, as does the politician, is that so often the short-term remedy conflicts with the long-term solution. Both have to accept, albeit with resignation, the limitations imposed by the structures on which they operate: the human body and the body politic. In consequence, the wisest course is often only a series of patching-up expedients. Careful research and observations can indicate worthwhile initiatives which are capable of ensuring that eventual benefits do accrue; but they may only rarely be dramatic or even directly attributable to their initiator. In an ideal world it would not sound horrifying, or cause alarm, if politicians and doctors admitted more freely and more openly that their decisions are often influenced and even dominated by the maxims of calculated neglect and masterly inactivity.

But while they know that this may be the wisest course, they also know that may be a course which opens them to bitter criticism, and in a crisis, to almost universal condemnation. Patients and parliaments want activism when faced with crisis.

In international politics calls for action are not new, as any reading of the reports from war correspondents from the Boer War and before will show. What is different today is the "CNN effect." The TV camera in Sarajevo recording minute by minute, hour by hour, day by day in real time from the battleground conveys an immediacy and has an impact that no newspaper, with its greater number of words qualifying and explaining, or even a radio commentary carries. While there is no CNN camera yet in the consulting room or operating theatre, medicine is now dramatised on TV and patients' rights and medical litigation have ensured that doctors no longer agonise in private when facing choices of life and death.

Doctors call this triage, the inescapable three-way choice, who to treat, who will die, who can wait. It is worth examining the qualities of the individual surgeon whom a doctor will choose for themselves or their family. One will invariably find that high up is a known reluctance to wield the scalpel for its own sake. This proper caution over intervening medically or surgically is as much about understanding the natural history of disease as recognising the dangers of upsetting the restorative nature of the body's defence mechanisms.

The general public has come to recognise even in the richest industrial nations that no system of public health care will provide wholly adequate resources. Some degree of rationing is accepted as inevitable, and this realization has heightened the question of how such choices should be made. As people realize that there will always be an unsatisfied medical demand, there is more questioning of whether rationing of facilities, or, more seriously, scarce medical and surgical skills—clear public goods – can be justified on anything other than the basis of need. But who determines that need, the doctors or the politicians? Since these subjective judgements are so complex we are finding it hard to escape from a mixed health care system, part publicly organized providing on the basis of need, part privately organized on the ability to pay.

A similar questioning is occurring within the international community about conflict prevention and resolution as it becomes ever clearer that we will not devote to it the much needed financial resources. We will defend our own State but are wary of involving our troops within another State's territory. In the early 1990s the Stockholm International Peace Research Institute showed that of 30 major armed conflicts in the world only one was interstate and that was between India and Pakistan. All the others were within States. Until the end of the Cold War the Security Council did not intervene in the internal affairs of a Member State. Now politicians and those who practice international diplomacy, after intervening in Iraq, Somalia and Bosnia-Herzegovina, are better aware of the perils of interventionism. As a result they are exhibiting a newfound sense of caution. In the US this caution manifested itself after Vietnam with the oft-repeated message that the US has no wish to become the world's policeman.

A new self-disciplined approach to UN intervention was first spelt out by President Clinton in a policy directive in April 1994, shortly after the last US troops left Somalia. The world was put on notice that the US believed that the Security Council could not respond to each and every crisis. Unfortunately, the Rwanda crisis in the spring of 1994 was the moment when the Security Council policy of accepting that the UN could not be everywhere or do everything, was first put to the test. The US refusal to sanction further UN involvement had been strongly influenced by what had happened in Somalia and what was happening in Bosnia-Herzegovina. Another strong and related motivation was Congressional resistance to paying for UN peacekeeping and a wish to control the spiraling US deficit in their assessed contribution to the UN budget. Yet in both Somalia and Bosnia-Herzegovina initially UN intervention saved hundreds of thousands of lives. In the autumn of 1992 both were seen as humanitarian interventions and so described but it was never going to be possible to keep such a limited mission beyond a few months. The international community should discard the illusion that one can intervene in a country beset by widespread civil violence without affecting domestic politics and without including a nation-building component.

The international community was under few illusions about the scale of the task if they were to intervene in Rwanda. They did know about the highly volatile ethnic composition of the country; of how the minority Tutsi had exercised economic and political domination prior to independence and how since independence in July 1962 the majority Hutu had ruled. Initially, Rwanda achieved modest economic growth (1.6% increase of GNP on average from 1965-1980). Even so, Rwanda had the highest population density in Africa and it was very vulnerable economically, with 80 per cent of its exports being coffee and tea. When the International Coffee Agreement collapsed in 1987 and the coffee price fell to half its 1980 value, we knew this would have a particularly damaging effect on Rwanda. It was then that conflict prevention in the form of economic assistance could have worked. We must examine the role of the Bretton Woods Institutions, the World Bank in particular, in any strategy for conflict prevention for the 21st Century.

In October 1990 an exiled Tutsi-dominated Rwandan Patriotic Front (RPF) attacked into north eastern Rwanda. The OAU organised a Neutral Military Observer Group

(NMOG) to monitor buffer zones separating the RPF and the Hutu Government forces in July 1992 and in February 1993 to ensure resettlement in demilitarized zones. In June 1993 the UN agreed to an Observer Mission into Uganda and Rwanda (UNAMUR) and it was sent in to implement a peace agreement concluded at Arusha in August 1993. The OAU lacked the resources among its Member States to carry through their political decision. In 1993 the UN Special Rapporteur observed that the situation was deteriorating with the Hutu Government labelling all the Tutsi people as accomplices of the RPF. Following the RPF invitation in 1990 France, sent its own soldiers and advisers. In October 1993 the United Nations Secretary General (UNSG) persuaded the Security Council to establish an Assistance Mission for Rwanda to help implement the Arusha Accords. By March 1994 UNAMIR's strength was 2,539 people with 24 participant countries. Then ten Belgian peacemakers were killed and the Belgian government announced they would withdraw. This dramatically changed the picture just as when 18 US Army Rangers lost their lives on 3–4 October 1993 in Somalia and US forces went on the defensive until their withdrawal on 31 March 1994. It seems that public opinion in many troop contributing countries will not accept such casualities from peacekeeping missions.

The Security Council then faced an all too familiar choice: to reinforce or to reduce the UN commitment. The Council chose to reduce. On 21 April, with the US in the lead, the UN Security Council decided to cut UNAMIR from 1,700 people to 270 people. This was done against the open advice of UN officials and all the main humanitarian NGOs operating in the country. By the end of April the aid agencies estimated that some 200,000 people had been killed in Rwanda. The killing rate rose thereafter remorselessly to over 500,000. On 13 May the UN Secretary General recommended that the

Security Council deploy 5,500 troops in an UNAMIR II. The US took the lead again within the Security Council in urging that UNAMIR II be confined to the borders of Rwanda and there was a slow buildup in troops. US officials were said to have been instructed by the State Department not to talk of acts of genocide so as to avoid incurring an obligation to act under the UN's Convention on Genocide. None of the governments on the Security Council could have been in any doubt that by then what was occurring was the largest and most explicit genocide the world had seen since the German genocide against the Jews.

Even so the Security Council was still not ready to deploy sufficient force to stop the Rwandan genocide and some doubted that even a large force could stop what was happening. Why were the permanent members so reluctant? In part, because it was happening on the African continent, which did not arouse as much public feeling as for example former Yugoslavia. In part, because in that part of the African continent, of the permanent members, only France had real interests. In part, because the Security Council felt that the Organisation of African Unity (OAU) and the surrounding African countries had neither the intention nor cohesion to participate in large numbers or the capacity to give much help for any large UN intervention from outside. The US felt they had been humiliated in Somalia. The French and British felt they were fully committed to peacekeeping in Bosnia. The Russians were otherwise engaged, not least in Chechnya. China had no links and was anyhow hostile to the very concept of intervention in the internal affairs of a Member State.

The world's press and TV covered the horror of what was happening extensively but there was never the same build up of public pressure to intervene as had happened over the famine in Ethiopia or was evident over the plight of the Kurds in 1991 and the humanitarian crisis in Somalia and Bosnia in 1992. It is easy, on moral grounds, to deplore the decision to limit UN intervention, but it was not a decision taken lightly or out of ignorance, but a decision bedded in realpolitik. Furthermore, it is the sort of decision which we can expect to be repeated.

Politicians should, therefore, take a leaf out of the medical profession's preventive discipline and institute a post mortem on the Rwanda genocide, a quite distinct investigation from the Rwanda War Crimes Tribunal. The findings of any such post mortem should examine the effect of the precipitate fall in the price of coffee in 1980 destabilising the Rwanda economy. People may rightly say that there are numerous other countries politically vulnerable to a fall in coffee price, but analysis may also show that of those countries few, if any, had the same combination of dependence on coffee exports and potential for ethnic instability.

A predictive capacity on potential conflicts is needed which is capable of reading across from economic to political factors. This cannot just be built up by the UN Secretary-General or the Security Council. Existing economic institutions who carefully and routinely monitor such factors must be mandated to work with the UN Secretary-General that should be charged with coordinating and publicly highlighting the implications of such research. Without a specific remit, the UN Secretary General will not get the involvement of institutions like the World Bank or International Monetary Fund who see themselves as totally separate from the UN in New York. Also any UN Secretary-General will be subjected to considerable pressure not to publish the findings for fear that it will be a self-fulfilling prophecy and the mere act of calling attention to a potential crisis will precipitate conflict.

Another area on which a Rwanda post mortem should focus is links established between the OAU and the UN as the OAU observer group was deployed. Could the observer group have been strengthened with some financial assistance or military logistic back-up and equipment? If this help could not come from the UN should this be the sort of specific action which the richer democracies should help finance? Could the economy of Rwanda have been buttressed at that time in 1992 with more international aid. We need to know exactly what financial help was asked for and what was refused.

Another issue that should be explored is if UN forces were never ready to be deployed in bulk, should they have gone in at all in 1993? Would it not have been wiser to have drawn the line not at increasing the size or the deployment pattern of an existing UN force, but at the concept of moving in at all, given the limitations and hesitations over further involvement? Politicians must not fail to look back on Rwanda, which has been the biggest single humanitarian disaster since the Second World War. If we do not learn lessons here there will be little hope for rational prevention and resolution of human conflict in the 21st Century.

Separate but similar post mortems are called for covering Bosnia-Herzegovina and Somalia. I have tried to contribute to this with an account of my own personal odyssey, but there are many other individuals concerned whose views should be tapped. The Carnegie Endowment Fund is sponsoring a Commission out of the Aspen Institute in Berlin to report in the summer of 1996 on the break up of the former Yugoslavia. The Security Council should commission a study on what disciplines can be adopted in future to curb the unreal nature of so many of the UN Security Council Resolutions. The World Bank should explore the Tito era and why the World Bank and other institutions lent so much money to Yugoslavia with so little conditionality. It is politically interesting why there was so little pressure for democratic reform in Yugoslavia.

Intellectuals were praising the dissident Djilas, but governments did little to reinforce his message.

In Somalia we need more retrospective analysis of the full extent of US involvement in all the military aspects of the peace-keeping exercise. This needs to be independently documented to counter the propaganda and scapegoating which has so far pushed all the blame on to the UN itself.

In the implementation of sanctions policy there is also much to be learnt from retrospective analysis. Sanctions against both Iraq and Serbia took a long time to bite on their regimes, during which time the effects on the civilian population were dire. A study published in *The Lancet* of 2 December 1995 on the health of Baghdad's children showed a strong association between economic sanctions and an increase in child mortality and malnutrition rates; the under five mortality rate rising five-fold. It claims that since August 1990 567,000 children in Iraq have died as a result of economic sanctions, which the Iraqi government refused to alleviate by exporting oil in exchange for food and medicine, denouncing this as an unacceptable interference in Iraqi sovereignty.

We need to examine carefully what financial measures and mechanisms are available to ensure a quicker impact on such governments and, if possible, where we can reduce the burden of sanctions on their civilian populations. President Mitterrand once remarked that the lesson of sanctions is that they are put on piecemeal, bite too slowly, and stay on too long. Sanctions against Serbia had their effect gravely weakened by the black market established with neighbouring countries.

One of the reasons why neighbouring governments did not clamp down on those black market activities was that their own economies were suffering serious damage and the UN Charter provision for alleviating the effect of sanctions on the surrounding areas was never invoked by the rich industrial nations. Oil and other goods flooded across from Macedonia and later Albania, to Serbia, rendering much of the work of the Sanctions Assistance Monitoring (SAMs) teams null and void.

One of the many reasons why sanctions are imposed in a haphazard way is that their application is often controversial within the Security Council and it is easier to apply them little by little, but we have to question whether this manner of implementation is not discrediting sanctions. Would the Security Council not be better off applying the discipline of an all or nothing approach to sanctions? There are humanitarian arguments for this line of thinking, for it appears that in Iraq and Serbia, hardship inflicted on innocent people was cumulative, hurting children and older people more as the years went on, while giving time for elites to develop a black market. Admittedly, the propaganda effect of sanctions was heightened by their governments wanting and ensuring bad publicity for the Security Council actions and using the suffering of their children in their battle with the rest of the world to have sanctions lifted.

There is an argument for moving to a strong full sanctions package immediately, and in particular, using financial sanctions at the start. For it appears that financial restrictions hurt governments more than their civilian population. We need, however, more evidence on this. We saw in 1986 that the actions of private banks in Switzerland in withholding credit from South Africa was a powerful factor in persuading the white South African regime to negotiate with the African National Congress and end apartheid. Had financial sanctions been used earlier in South Africa there might not have been the 13 year period between the first mandatory sanctions on arms being applied in 1977 and opening of the path to negotiations in 1990. Financial sanctions can have their effectiveness massively enhanced by the legislative powers member States took in the

1980s to monitor and control drug money. It is now very hard for any government to evade the seizure of their financial assets. It was noticeable that the threat of financial sanctions, to take effect at the end of April 1993, was the key factor in convincing President Milosevic to accept the Vance-Owen Peace Plan.

Just as a little medicine can have no curative value, so a minimalist sanctions package can often have little damaging effect on the economy of a country and can even, as we saw in Rhodesia in the 1960s and early 1970s, by encouraging import substitution and self-sufficiency, bolster economic performance in the medium term. The world needs to consider these factors very carefully before embarking on any new sanctions strategy. It has been noticeable that, for example, over Nigeria there has been much heart-searching and serious questioning of the effects. Sanctions must not be imposed just to satisfy public opinion in Security Council countries. A maritime or land based blockade of all goods has to be counter balanced by food aid and medical supplies best supplied from the start by UNHCR and WHO. Inevitably much of such food aid will feed the armies. By 1995 it was estimated that more than 50 percent of the food going into Bosnia-Herzegovina went to feed the three armies and it was also continuously traded on the black market.

The other self-discipline that needs to be applied relates to the differing forms of military intervention. It is not an easy area to establish clarity, but politicians should perhaps again learn a lesson from the therapeutic application of poisons and radiotherapy in the treatment of cancer. Military intervention will always be a dangerous operation; even more so if the task of peacekeeping has any elements of enforcement. The UN has developed special peacekeeping techniques for monitoring and observing ceasefire agreements. The parties to a dispute have to be agreed on the UN force coming in, and what the UN forces' main tasks are before it arrives in the area. We need to recognise that there is no such thing as a surgical intervention in a civil war. The arrival of any external military force will change the dynamics of that war. If it is announced in advance that the force will only stay for six weeks or a few months then the parties may only play for time until the force exits. Limitations on the force can easily encourage one or other of the fighting parties to await withdrawal. It is also unwise to spell out to the fighting parties that the intervening forces will never impose a settlement. In both Somalia and Bosnia-Herzegovina the parties soon knew that the UN would not impose a settlement and, for much of the time, felt they might leave. While an exit strategy for the UN is often thought by troop-contributing countries to be essential, usually the less it can be talked about the better. Timetables may concentrate minds, but not always in the most helpful way.

Can there ever be a purely humanitarian intervention? After the experience of the humanitarian military intervention in Bosnia-Herzegovina, there will be a legacy of hostility within the Security Council to believing that such an exercise, with its initial restrictive mandate, can ever be repeated. Their scepticism is understandable but regrettable. In terms of lives saved, either from malnutrition or hypothermia, during the winter of 1992-93, the Bosnian humanitarian operation was an unqualified success. Its restricted mandate worked for the first few months and became impossible only after the Bosnian Serbs had rejected the Vance/Owen, UN/EU Peace Plan. That was the time, as I argued, at the end of May 1993, to have withdrawn the UN forces from exposed ground and used NATO air power to impose a settlement which NATO would then have had to implement.

Over two years later in September 1995, that is in effect what was done. But by then the ethnic cleansing had continued at such a rate that partition was all that was left. The lesson is that a strictly humanitarian intervention can probably only be sustained for six months or a year. Humanitarian interventions depend absolutely on the UN forces being seen at all times acting impartially. Peacekeeping is greatly helped if one is able to rely on the cooperation of all the parties. But in the absence of being able to act impartially, then a strictly humanitarian intervention becomes unsustainable. Also, if the Security Council cannot maintain the self-discipline to be impartial it is better not to launch a strictly humanitarian intervention, for that will undermine the credibility of the force. Nation-building, and restoring civil order takes years, not months, and can necessitate fairly large force levels. To conduct oneself with impartiality is not the same as being neutral. UN commanders must be free to criticise abuses and to authorise their forces to fire back when fired on.

Another limiting factor is that military intervention to peace-keep, to peace-enforce, or to assist humanitarian relief will involve casualties and troop-contributing countries must be able to carry public opinion in their own countries when faced by such an eventuality. Troop contributing countries must also be able to influence Security Council resolutions to ensure they are based on the realities on the ground. For all these reasons Security Council Member States should be obliged to make an effective contribution to a UN Rapid Reaction Force during their time as members of the Council. In that way rhetoric and reality may be matched better than at present. Since UN interventions fail where rhetoric bears little relation to reality. In all cases of UN intervention we have, as part of the price of rapid deployment, to be ready to cut one's losses and leave. Intervention cannot always be sustained and knowing when to leave is as important as knowing when to enter.

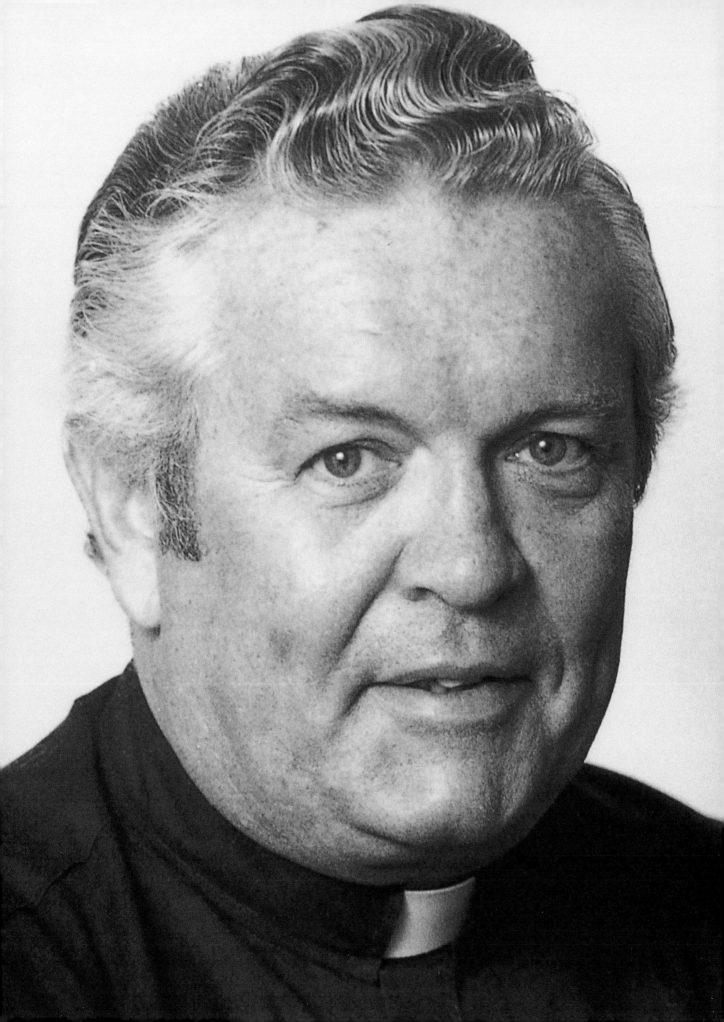

Aengus Finucane

*His Distinguished International Lecture was delivered
in the College on September 28, 1992*

Aengus Finucane, C.S.Sp., was a missionary
priest in Nigeria during the Biafran war in the
late 1960's. During that disaster, he founded
Africa Concern; this charity evolved into an
international organization, Concern Worldwide,
alleviating hunger, famine, and serving refugee
communities in over 50 countries with a
multimillion dollar budget and thousands of
field workers. Father Finucane worked in disaster
zones in Uganda, Bangladesh, Somalia, and
on the Thai-Cambodian border. He received
honorary doctorates from several universities,
and was awarded the "Freedom of the City" by
his native Limerick in Ireland. He died in 2009.

The Changing Roles of Voluntary Organizations
Aengus Finucane

I was parish priest of Uli, Nigeria, in 1968. It was there during the Biafra/Nigeria civil war, that I had my first experience in the delivery of humanitarian aid and health services under conflict conditions. The eastern region of Nigeria had seceded as Biafra, and the federal Nigerian government was sparing no effort to reintegrate the oil-rich breakaway region. Uli, a rural townland deep in Biafra, became the epicenter of a massive relief operation. The road just outside my parish residence was widened to make an airstrip. All flying was at night and the planes had to run the gauntlet of the federal Nigerian forces. With vastly superior firepower, they were steadily squeezing and reducing Biafran-held territory. "Uli Airport" found a place on the world map. By October 1968 it had become the busiest airport in Africa: On some nights it handled as many as fifty planes. My parish church became a feeding center. Sermons were exhortations to eat mice, cockroaches, and cassava leaves. Parish duties gave way to airport duties.

In the final months of the Biafra/Nigeria conflict in late 1969 I was based in Libreville, Gabon. From there I was organizing the airlift of relief supplies to Uli for Concern, a newly formed Irish relief organization. Having unloaded their relief cargoes at Uli, the returning planes brought thousands of near-dead children to be cared for by non-governmental organizations (NGOs) in camps set up for them in neighbouring countries.

More than twenty years later, in August 1992, I flew into Baidoa, a famine-stricken town of 60,000 people in Somalia. I was on board a cargo plane carrying sixteen tons of supplies for a Concern relief team. In Somalia on the opposite side of Africa from Biafra, another chapter of misery, tragedy and famine was unfolding. Prior to this famine, Baidoa had been as little known to the outside world as Uli had been before the Biafra conflict. In August 1992, television, radio and print media in Baidoa catapulted the town into the center of the world stage. In the days I was there, the satellite dishes and elaborate equipment of two television groups beamed the misery and dying of Baidoa into living-rooms around the world.

During the time of that visit to Baidoa, an average of two hundred deaths were recorded daily. On one day trucks collected 176 corpses for burial. These were the bodies of people with no friends to bury them. Most often the near-dead buried their dead in shallow graves. The population swelled as more and more starving people were drawn to the town. In the first ten days of September 1992, the trucks collected 2,353 bodies from the streets of Baidoa, and 70 per cent of them were children. By September 16th, the grim tally had reached 3,520!

NGO Origins and Growth

Uli to Baidoa; Biafra to Somalia: 1968–1992. A huge proliferation and wide diversification of NGOs took place during these years. It is little short of obscene that two such gruesome landmarks as Uli and Baidoa stand as the parameters for this personal record of relief work.

There were NGOs before Biafra. But NGOs in the sense we know them today—as accepted players with a major role in the transfer of resources from rich to poor countries only became a prominent force on the multinational Third World aid stage in the 1970's and the 1980's. The whole concept of Third World development through the transfer of resources from richer to poorer countries belongs to the post-colonial era of the second half of this century. The international Third World NGOs we now know are, in a few instances, a development of older organizations. For example, Save the Children, UK., have roots going back to 1919 and a shattered post-World War I in Europe. Oxfam was formed in England in 1943 to help children in Belgium and Greece during World War II. CARE was formed in the United States to send relief parcels to post-World War II Europe.

Early NGOs were driven by a Western and Christian philosophy of caring for the needy. Church founded or "confessional NGOs" only developed from the 1950's onwards. Their core constituency consists of their church membership. Although they run parallel to church structures, they are usually at great pains to keep their development and relief work separate from their religious or evangelistic work. They make considerable efforts to ensure that their work is targeted on the most needy, regardless of their religious affiliation, and in ways calculated to benefit the population in general. The past thirty years have also seen the emergence of many non-aligned NGOs on the international stage. While the majority are non-denominational and secular, they are still inspired by the same Western philosophy of caring that motivated the earlier NGOs.

There are countless non-profit organizations and groups that are non-governmental which quite justifiably describe themselves as NGOs. However, tonight I am concerned only with the international NGOs that have as their sole or prime purpose the righting of the imbalance between rich and poor countries by the transfer of resources. Some of these NGOs deal exclusively with children, or with crisis interventions, or health or agriculture. Some NGOs confine their efforts to fund-raising or the mobilization of resources such as pharmaceuticals and hospital supplies for developing countries. Others concentrate on development education or lobbying on behalf of developing countries.

As we approach the millennium, lines between the forms of activity pursued by NGOs are becoming increasingly blurred. The greater complexity of needs sometimes pushes organizations toward specialization and the development of high levels of expertise. Some other organizations are pressured, in order to the maintain or increase levels of funding, toward diversification in order to be able to provide a wider range of choices to funders.

There is a major distinction between organizations which directly manage and implement projects in developing countries and organizations which confine themselves to raising funds or mobilizing resources for transfer to operational partners. Voluntary organizations frequently come under pressure from supporters to address domestic needs.

The Effect of Biafra on NGOs

Third World NGOs came into their own during the involvement in Biafra. Biafra created a new level of awareness of Third World famine and disaster in the West. It was the first major disaster that was brought into the living rooms of the world by television, which, with its visual immediacy, challenged indifference to faraway suffering.

The Biafrans fought a good propaganda war. They engaged Mark Press, a Geneva based public relations firm, to present their case to the world. The Biafrans used the sufferings of their people to great effect to disturb the world consciences. In Biafra, the many NGOs involved also learned the usefulness of the media, a lesson that has stood them in good stead in winning support for their work ever since. The response to Biafra demonstrated that people do care; obtaining support is a question of getting the message to them. Since Biafra, NGOs are very conscious of their responsibility to inform the world of disasters and suffering so that the problem may be addressed. The "confessional" NGOs were the most active in Biafra. The Protestant organizations were grouped under the World Council of Churches (WCC), and the Catholic NGOs were grouped under Caritas. Together they formed a strong and influential operational body, Joint Church Aid (JCA), which was also substantially funded by the American Jewish Committee. It was an unprecedented example of co-operation between world religious bodies. Dozens of private agencies from twenty countries grouped together under the JCA banner. JCA funded and ran a huge airlift to beleaguered Biafra, a lifeline that linked into the extensive church networks on the ground and became a highly effective distribution system for the supplies being airlifted to the country by the international NGOs and other donors. In western countries NGOs which were not themselves operational joined Joint Church Aid and supported the relief efforts by donating to JCA.

New NGOs were formed in response to the needs in Biafra. Concern and Medicins Sans Frontiers are two such organizations. Others, such as Canair Relief, were operational during the crisis then disbanded, and in the mid 1980's Band Aid made a similar appearance in response to famine needs in Ethiopia and Sudan and then disbanded. After the Biafran crisis Concern debated disbanding. However, the Bangladesh crisis of 1971 decided the question in favour of continuing.

The new and extraordinary role of NGOs in Biafra proved that there was indeed a niche and a role for NGOs in the international stage. In Biafra, NGOs discovered that they had particular strengths in emergency situations, and ever since then they have played a prominent role in virtually every disaster relief operation. NGOs have become a great deal more professional and sophisticated. Many of the organizations that are now operational in disaster relief situations have become particularly effective in delivering health services and humanitarian assistance.

The biggest change in NGOs during the past thirty years have been an increase in size. Several grew into multi-million dollar operations. Even some of the smaller ones most frequently active in conflict and disaster situations now have annual budgets of forty to fifty million dollars. It is difficult to operate on a small budget in disaster situations. In some of the major disaster situations of the 1990's, as in Liberia and Somalia, government services scarcely functioned. When governments break down, UN Agencies, which usually operate through governments, are severely hampered. In such situations NGOs which have not developed their own back-up systems are also left adrift.

Idealism and humanitarianism were undoubtedly the forces which gave birth to many of the international NGOs. In the case of the "confessional" NGOs, a religious motivation was added. Many organizations had charismatic founder members. Growth in scale inevitably meant organizations became less personalized. Although the general public still looks on the operatives in the NGOs as ill paid or even unpaid, and highly idealistic, most people might be somewhat shocked if they saw the salary and operating budgets of major, and even smaller, NGOs. While most NGOs are very cost conscious, they are repeatedly confronted with the "pay peanuts and get monkeys" dilemma. To get the kind of high-level, professionally qualified personnel necessary to handle the complexities if large organizations cost money. Being entrusted with huge resources by the public and by governments and institutions imposes great responsibilities.

In Biafra, NGOs were effective and highly successful largely because there was an extensive network of professional, committed personnel already in place. No disaster, especially no disaster in a conflict situation, has since enjoyed that luxury. In Somalia, twenty-five years later, there were virtually no ready-made feed-in points with which NGOs could connect. Among the operational agencies, those with their own backup systems stood by far the best chance of doing extensive and effective work. It was distressing to see NGOs abounding in goodwill floundering because of lack of support systems.

The JCA airlift into Biafra has never been fully recognized for what it was. Recalling it now helps put the belated and pathetic efforts to get assistance to Somalia in perspective. Many of the JCA planes carried fifteen tons per flight to Uli, and it was a major disappointment if each plane did not manage two flights each night. And they were operating by night under constant threat of Federal Nigerian fire. At the height of the conflict JCA handled 376 tons of relief supplies in a single night at Uli. Although there was a cease-fire in Somalia in 1992, and Baidoa has a very good airstrip, two large U.S. Air Force planes were each making one trip a day from Mombassa to Baidoa and each carrying but nine tons of supplies.

Where there is a will, there is a way. There was a will in Biafra. Twenty-five years later, there wasn't a will in Somalia until very late in the game, and even then it was lukewarm for too long. One can only be cynical about the uncoordinated efforts of the superpowers in Somalia. In the years since Biafra we had launched satellites into space, put people on the moon, and made all manner of technological advances. At the end of July 1992, there were twenty-five million metric tons of cereal in European intervention stores alone. Given these facts, how did the world community cope with the shame of watching hundreds of thousands of people die of starvation? It was not that we did not know.

There is an ever-present danger that NGOs may become overconfident because of their undoubted success in small undertakings. They often overstretch themselves, but they should stretch themselves. They can also annoy other actors on the stage by raising strident voices and finger-pointing, by exaggerating their own expertise and capabilities, by seeming to lay claim to a monopoly on caring. Such actions can build up unreal expectations. Often because of their own frustration and inability to deliver, bigger actors have lured NGOs out of their depth. The NGOs can be like small fishing trawlers tempted into deep waters to service large factory ships. Usually they respond with alacrity. When the factory ships fail to function, the smaller vessels are in dire trouble.

NGOs are but one actor, and usually a relatively small one, on the international aid stage. This should be borne in mind especially in conflict situations. They must function in an awareness of, and with respect for, bilateral, or government donors, multilateral donors, host government and, where they are present, local NGOs. Whether in conflict, disaster, or long-term work situations, NGOs should respect local institutions, culture and customs. Far too often many NGO personnel display a staggering lack of sensitivity and respect for their host environment.

Government to Government Aid

During the last thirty years there has been a growing disillusionment among donor governments with regard to recipient Third World partner governments. Unreal expectations have been replaced with often bitter recriminations. In reviewing government to government, or bilateral aid, it should be borne in mind that seldom was such aid purely altruistic.

Most bilateral aid is in large part motivated by self interest, by political, commercial, and strategic considerations. Prime Minister of Great Britain, Margaret Thatcher was noted for putting things bluntly; she stated very simply that "British Aid must foster British Trade."

Through the 1980's and into the early nineties, bilateral donors, as already noted, channelled increasing amounts of aid through international NGOs. This was sometimes resented by Third World governments. They resented being by-passed and seemingly not trusted. I noted such reactions when dealing with officials in Ethiopia, Sudan and Bangladesh.

The government of newly independent Eritrea took a strong stand against the involvement of international NGOs, and of UN agencies, in the delivery of aid. The Eritreans were the ones who most strongly voiced feelings increasingly shared by other Third World governments. They were prepared to accept the consequent reduction in aid flows. This more independent line is gaining strength in the emerging African political bloc made up of Eritrea, Ethiopia, Uganda and Rwanda. This bloc enjoys the sympathies of Tanzania, Zambia, Zimbabwe and Burundi.

The sometimes startling growth in size of the international NGOs in the 1980's and 1990's is largely attributable to the partnership with donor governments in the transfer of aid. The growth in size too often entailed an erosion of ethos which went hand in hand with the replacement of committed volunteerism and low paid service by costly professionalism which the more complex organizations required. More fundamentally, increased government funding of NGO work entails a lessening of the independence of the NGOs. This is, of course, particularly likely if an NGO becomes heavily dependent on a single government source. NGOs must be careful not to become the tools or simply the contractors of donor governments. At the same time, NGOs are committed to exploiting to the fullest all resource possibilities on behalf of their clients, and government resources offer the greatest possibility. Availing of government resources to the fullest while retaining independence and remaining true to the ethos can be very difficult.

The scale of fund-raising necessary to maintain the larger NGOs has fostered many well oiled NGO publicity and lobbying machines. Sadly the growth and increased efficiency on the public relations and fund-raising side of the NGOs has too often not been matched by a proportionate improved performance, and has been accompanied by some sacrificing of independence. Bigger is by no means necessarily better.

Lobbying is a vitally important role that some NGOs specialize in, and all NGOs exercise at times. For a year, while Somalia drifted ever faster toward anarchy, the country was not on the world agenda. Individual NGOs and NGO networks, which now exist in considerable numbers, worked hard to publicize Somalia's plight. Media personnel were encouraged to visit Somalia and were facilitated in every way. Once interest is nurtured to a certain point, it snowballs, feeding on itself.

Politicians and governments were lobbied at the same time as the public. As the wave of public concern for Somalia grew, so too did politicians' awareness. Many, somewhat belatedly, showed an interest. In major disasters and conflict situations the intervention of governments is critical in addressing the large-scale needs. Involving governments is a role NGOs can play. NGOs can blaze an action trail on the ground, but their resources, even when augmented by bilateral and multilateral inputs, cannot cope with disasters on a grand scale. The sooner governments become openly interested the better.

Some donor governments have shown preference for local or national organizations over international NGOs as operational partners in the distribution of aid. International donors, notably Britain, the United States and the European Union, have strengthened their field offices in tandem with this policy shift. International NGOs which had expanded through the eighties on the strength of government funding have sometimes found themselves with spare capacity. Some have retrenched. Many have seriously reviewed their strategies. Increasingly they, like the bilateral donors, are entering into partnerships with local or national groups in their countries of operation. While governments in the somewhat more stable developing countries can lay down stringent conditions for the aid donors, and aid donors can find seemingly suitable operational partners in these countries, there are many poor countries which can not afford this stance where local partners are not available.

In most developing countries when a major disaster strikes or there is a major population upheaval because of conflict, it is unlikely that services adequate in peace time will be able to cope. The scope and need for international NGOs in these circumstances continues to be enormous. At such times recipient governments are open to offers of assistance and their bilateral donors are glad to support international NGOs. Somalia was a good example of this.

Bilaterals in Somalia

The slowness of governments in responding to non strategic tragedies was illustrated in Somalia. In August 1992, Ireland's David Andrews became, the first foreign minister to visit famine ravished Somalia. He went at the invitation of NGOs and was shocked into action by what he saw. He immediately contacted all European Community foreign ministers and the UN. The British, the Dutch, and the Germans responded immediately with increased aid. The US initiative followed shortly thereafter. Also at this time Boutros Boutros-Ghali,

Secretary General of the United Nations, ruffled many feathers by accusing the world community of neglecting the poor man's plight in Africa while paying great attention to the rich man's war in former Yugoslavia.

Some governments, notably the British, had been supportive of NGOs before, but it was only when other governments became openly involved that things began to move. For many, however, it was too late. It should be remembered that the tragedy of Somalia was enacted against the backdrop of world leaders gathered in Rio de Janeiro for the United Nations World Environmental Conference. The international chorus singing about a better world order in Rio was sadly out of tune with, and seemingly unaware of, the suffering in Somalia.

Funding relationships between donor governments and NGOs are highly important and useful to both parties in the delivery of services in disasters. Acting through NGOs enables donor governments to follow their consciences in transferring resources, even if they have grave reservations about the local government and do not wish to support it. They can bypass (to an extent) governments of which they disapprove and reach the "deserving poor."

For all kinds of reasons, governments may be less generous to some recipient countries than for others. There can be very definite political discrimination in the distribution of aid. This was particularly so during the Cold War. Ethiopia and Cambodia were ruled out by many Western countries for development aid. This criterion is, however, applied rather selectively. The tyrant Siad Barre was supported in Somalia for strategic reasons. If a clean human rights record was made an essential criterion for receiving aid, there would be a very short recipient list.

Humanitarian aid, however, is treated differently than so-called development aid by donors. There is vastly less self-interest or hidden political agendas attached. Donor governments may channel such aid through NGOs to movements they do not officially recognize as having legal status while they continue to recognize the de facto government. Eritrea and Tigray within Mengistu's Ethiopia are good examples of this.

The Multilateral Organizations

Despite their shortcomings, the multilaterals, especially the UN specialized agencies and the EC are close and supportive forces for the NGOs in the Third World activities. In normal operating circumstances they are geared to longer-term work, and they can be slow off the mark in disaster situations. Many field offices become comfortable and complacent. Like many others – bilaterals and NGOs included – they are loathe to move from development to relief or emergency work.

There are two dangers in analyzing the performance of any of the actors on the stage in disaster situations. One is to flail out and condemn the people on the ground doing the work, which is a bit like shooting the messenger. The other danger is of closing ranks and covering up – sweeping the death statistics under the carpet. An agency's operations are only as good as they are allowed to be by those who direct them. Operatives of UN Agencies tend to be smothered by bureaucratic requirements; their flexibility is stifled. They cannot indulge the kind of gut reactions that are necessary to save lives in disasters.

NGOs too, in growing and handling very large budgets, can become very high handed and excessively bureaucratic. As they grow they tend to lose their flexibility and spontaneity. They become more and more like the multilateral and bilateral agencies that they criticize. They should learn from what happened to the bigger actors in Somalia. A permanent UN co-ordinating agency with the muscle to be effective is certainly needed. This body should include teams which can be deployed to disaster situations. One of the greatest tragedies of disaster situations is the lack of experienced workers. The sight of a new generation sadly reinventing the wheel is common when disasters strike.

Local Relief Structures

Normally, national and local government must be the principal actors in disaster situations. There are exceptions, such as Somalia, where there was literally no government through 1992. In most disaster situations there is some developed services structure. While some such structures are quite sophisticated, in most countries in the Third World, health and humanitarian services are altogether inadequate even in normal times. There is no way they can cope alone with the massively expanded demands that arise in a major disaster. Neither is it likely that they will have the capacity to utilize quickly and effectively the resources handed over to them. Local governments are very unlikely to accept this reality. They are generally, and understandably, slow to admit to any weakness.

Host governments should be respected. Unfortunately there may come a point where, for humanitarian reasons, government and government regulations should be circumvented. It is important to consider the role of local NGOs which are funded by international donors. There has been a proliferation of non-governmental organizations in developing countries because of the development of foreign aid during the last twenty to thirty years. These organizations depend for their existence on being part of the delivery of international aid within their own countries. For the most part, unlike the international NGOs, they do not raise funds by soliciting donations for their work within their own countries.

Many international NGOs have devoted considerable effort to fostering the growth of local NGOs. Quite often the local

NGOs were set up as partners linked to the principal. This has particularly been the case with "confessional" NGOs. Parent churches which had earlier developed local counterpart churches have formed development sections for the transfer of material aid to developing countries. They have supported local churches in developing parallel recipient aid sections.

Besides the "confessional" NGOs linked to churches, purely secular NGOs dependent on international funding have emerged. Large amounts of international aid, sometimes amounting to millions of dollars annually, have been channelled through them. Some of these NGOs are highly sophisticated and operate on a grand scale. However, as with the international NGOs, they are vulnerable to the hazards of growth.

Many developing countries afford a poor climate for the development of local NGOs, especially for NGOs with international linkages. Few developing countries have real democratic governments. Many are under military rule or are governed by a one party system. NGOs are unlikely to enjoy a great deal of freedom. There is a desperate desire on the part of some international NGOs, shared by theorists and increasingly by major funders, to demonstrate a high level of local NGO participation in the delivery of aid. The international development literature portrays a very inflated image of local NGOs.

The freedom of speech and action which is enjoyed by NGOs in western democracies is presumed to obtain in developing countries. However, freedom of action and association is very limited in many Third World countries. The local NGOs which can maintain strong international links stand the best chance of surviving. The reality is that there isn't a great body of independent and genuinely local NGOs in the Third World. They will undoubtedly play an ever greater role in long term development. However, they are unlikely to be major players in disaster and conflict situations in the foreseeable future.

The development of national NGOs in the developing countries will have a major bearing on the future role of the international NGOs. They will still have a role but a lessening one within the more stable and democratic developing countries. The local NGOs as the preferred partners of donor governments and, being more acceptable to their own governments, will assume an ever greater role on the international aid stage in these countries. Very many developing countries, especially in Africa, do not provide the environment for the development of strong local NGOs. In these countries there will, for many years to come, be room for a very significant international NGO input in development as well at times of natural disasters.

In times of conflict, of major population upheavals and refugee movements, the international donor community will, for the foreseeable future, continue to depend on the international NGOs to provide much of the last link in the chain of response. The private donors in western countries are most likely to continue to entrust their giving to the international NGOs. The personalized response of caring individuals to world poverty and disaster needs will continue to seek a channel other than official government channels. The international NGOs will also continue to be a conduit for some of the official aid from their own countries.

In a world where 1.3 billion people survive on less than the equivalent of a $1 a day, where nearly a billion are illiterate; some 840 million go hungry or face food insecurity, and nearly a third of the people in the least developed countries – most of them in sub Saharan Africa – are not expected to survive to age 40, the need for international NGOs is greater than ever. They are adapting and adjusting to circumstances. This they must continue to do. They must not question their relevance.

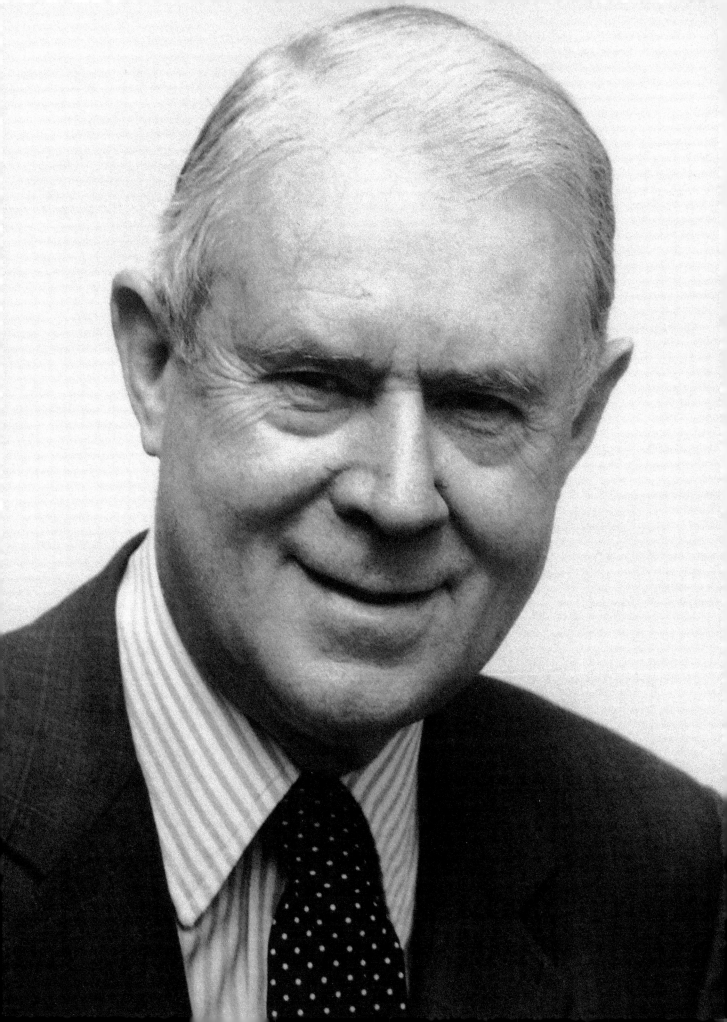

Cyrus R. Vance

His Distinguished International Lecture was delivered in the College on October 1, 1991.

In the United States of America, Cyrus R. Vance was, arguably, the most respected public figure in the last part of the 20th century. He served as Secretary of the Army, Deputy Secretary of Defense and Secretary of State. His integrity and diplomatic skills were used by the United States and the United Nations in a wide variety of crises including those in Korea, Dominican Republic, Cyprus, South Africa, and the Former Yugoslavia. He received the highest civilian award of his own country, the Presidential Medal of Freedom, and those of England, France, and Japan. Once, after meeting with one of my medical school classes, he noted that he had never considered the potential role of health and humanitarian efforts as tools in diplomacy. This observation led to the founding of The Center for International Humanitarian Cooperation (CIHC), and he remained a Director of the Center till his death in 2002.

Meeting the Challenges of the New Millennium
Cyrus Vance

As we approach a new millennium, scores of people began offering definitions of what has been called a "new world order." A number of them seem to have in mind only enhanced collective military security.

For my part, I am convinced that a "new world order" cannot be confined to questions of military security, nor can it be based on notions of the United States as world arbiter.

In that spirit, and recognizing that the world situation impels us to look for solutions that might have been previously impossible, let me offer a few suggestions.

I propose them as challenges for us to rise to as we move through space and time to keep our date with the millennial year 2000. A new world order for the twenty-first century, I believe, should be structured along the general lines of the 1991 Stockholm Initiative to meet the following six imperatives:

1) International peace and security
2) Sustainable economic development
3) Curbing uncontrolled population growth and environmental degradation
4) Providing adequate global health care
5) Fostering democracy and human rights
6) Strengthening key international institutions

International Peace and Security

The first and primary imperative of a new world order must be the maintenance of peace and security on both a global and a regional scale.

Although the Cold War may be over, we need to look no further than the nightly television news to recognize that national, ethnic, religious, and other conflicts – both across and inside national borders – continue to pose grave threats to peace and security.

The disintegration of Yugoslavia into bitter civil war tragically demonstrates how real and destructive these conflicts can be. The dissolution of the former Soviet Union contains serious flash points – some of which have already led to conflict. Other potential flash points also exist in Eastern and Central Europe. Nor is ethnic and religious conflict limited to Europe. We must never forget, nor can the world ignore, similar violence in Somalia, Angola, Liberia and other parts of Africa, Central Asia, and the Indian subcontinent. In short, the end of the Cold War has by no means brought an end to violence and conflict on our planet.

Beyond maintaining appropriate military capabilities, we should begin our search for peace and greater security by strengthening the mandate and the capabilities of the institution that has the widest and potentially most effective reach – the United Nations.

The UN's collective security potential was demonstrated during the Gulf crisis. After Iraq's invasion of Kuwait, nations working within the UN framework impressively and effectively applied an unprecedented policy of embargo, containment, and enforcement. And when the war ended, there was no choice but to turn increasingly to the United Nations to provide long-term stability and humanitarian aid.

Yet, with new thinking in mind, imagine for a moment what might have been possible had the UN at the time of the Gulf War possessed the capability to head off Iraq's aggression.

In this connection, Prime Minister Ingvar Carlsson's Stockholm Initiative recommends the establishment of a global emergency system within the United Nations. This proposal has been reinforced by UN Secretary General Boutros Boutros-Ghali in "An Agenda for Peace."

Under this proposal, which I support, UN political offices would be established *inter alia* in key locations, such as Iraq/Kuwait and South Korea/North Korea, to provide early warning of potential aggression and thus, it is hoped, deter potential conflict. But that alone would be inadequate. The UN also needs its own collective security forces – by which I mean earmarked forces that would be available on the call of the Security Council – to intervene when the Security Council so determines.

To make the global emergency system effective, the Secretary-General should be granted greater lee-way to deploy the organization's diplomatic, monitoring, and dispute-resolution capabilities whenever requested by a member state.

A UN with such capacity and authority could have posted buffer forces on the Iraq-Kuwait border could have facilitated early peaceful discussion of the two countries' border disputes, and could have signaled clearly that Iraqi aggression would almost certainly trigger a collective response by the world community.

But the United Nations cannot be everywhere. To keep the peace, we also need to modernize regional security arrangements, particularly in volatile areas like the Middle East, the Horn of Africa, and South Asia, where no effective regional institutions now exist.

The Conference on Security and Cooperation in Europe – known as CSCE – has facilitated to a degree the post-Cold War thaw that is taking place in Central and parts of Eastern Europe. The North Atlantic Treaty Organization was the Western shield that kept a fragile situation stable until a thaw could take place. But it was CSCE, through treaties and confidence-building measures, that helped the former Soviet Union and Central and Eastern European countries to begin to work their way to democracy and free-market economies. But much more remains to be done.

As the Middle East peace process moves painstakingly forward, the CSCE model should be considered. Obviously, on one level, the meetings now under way are discussing Arab-Israeli relations and the issue of a Palestinian homeland. On another level, affected nations both inside and outside the region are beginning to tackle a broader range of issues, including regional security arrangements, human rights, environmental degradation, refugees, economic cooperation, and restraints on the development and transfer of all kinds of weapons.

As to the last of these, there is a crying need to rid the Middle East of all weapons of mass destruction and methods of their delivery as soon as possible. The radical limitation of conventional arms exports to the Middle East must also be addressed as a matter of top priority.

In the United States we regard it as quite normal that we should be beginning to reduce strategic weapons and other military expenditures, and to re-allocate the resources to domestic priorities. Yet in the Middle East and much of the rest of the world, arms sales continue minimally abated. Unfortunately, the United States and other arms-exporting nations persist in viewing such transfers as commercial opportunities rather than potential threats to regional and, as we have seen, our own security. We urgently need a convention limiting the sale of conventional arms, especially in the Middle East.

Sustainable Economic Development

Correspondingly, peace and development will be served if a prospective new world order includes a recommitment to international economic cooperation and increased development assistance.

Both the United States and other countries have had bouts of protectionist flu as economic pressures and changing world trading patterns have endangered the previous worldwide consensus on access to goods and money.

President Kennedy, when he signed the historic Trade Expansion Act of 1962, remarked that "a rising tide lifts all boats." The premise remains true, but sadly, its support is less widespread than one would hope.

The General Agreement on Tariffs and Trade (GATT) needs to be reinforced, not weakened, as seems to be the drift today. When the International Monetary Fund (IMF) and World Bank were created at Bretton Woods, the GATT was seen as the global trade organization that could accommodate the interests of both developed and developing countries, while holding back the protectionist and mercantilist forces that were so destructive in the past. But protectionist forces now seem, unfortunately, to be gaining strength, rather than waning.

The GATT, World Bank, IMF, and UNCTAD—the UN Conference on Trade and Development—all are important global institutions. They are complemented by regional trade and financial entities such as the European Community; the Asian, African, and Latin American development banks; and the European Bank for Reconstruction and Development. Regional groups have taken on new life. That is good. But it would be tragic for all of us if this were to end up dividing the world into European, Asian, and North American economic blocs pitted against each other, while leaving the world's poor nations on the outside looking in.

Have-not nations cannot prosper absent a free and open international economic and financial environment. But such an environment alone will not ensure sustained growth. No viable new world order can be based on a trickle-down theory.

We must not forget, however, that the history of the past fifty years has shown us a number of surprising economic success stories. The development process, once begun, takes on a dynamic momentum that carries it forward at a self-sustaining rate. Certain interrelated factors can be identified as reasons for success: investments in human capital through better education, health care, population planning, and training; investments in infrastructure and industry that have the long-term prospect of bringing success in international markets; development of domestic agricultural production, distribution, and processing

By the same token, we have learned that grandiose projects such as dams, superhighways, steel mills, and modern airport complexes often do not make sense unless they are part of sound, overall plans for sustainable economic development.

We must face the dual realities that slow growth in both developed and developing nations illustrates a downside of interdependence: namely, that slow growth in each diminishes demands for products of the other. Similarly, we must also recognize that debt service continues to consume a major share of developing country resources. Even resource-rich but heavily indebted potential powerhouses such as Brazil will do well in the next decade not to lose ground. And it is evident that these issues are severely aggravated by problems of populations, environment, and refugees.

The common thread that links these complex intersecting factors is evident: no nation can resolve all its own problems without the help of other nations. Common action and common security are essential. We have learned from hard experiences that multilateral global action is the only way we can achieve widespread sustainable economic growth and expanding investment.

The United Nations estimates that one billion people – one-fifth of the world population – now live in extreme poverty. Yet the World Bank estimates that with sufficient investment, this number could be reduced by almost half by the end of the decade. Such an effort would require that all nations commit themselves to simple and discrete targets.

The worldwide cost of meeting key social development targets is estimated at $20 billion annually – the cost of sustaining the Gulf War for a fortnight. It is all a question of priorities: Do we care enough to make a similar investment in the future of humanity?

The long-cited target for development assistance is that each industrialized country provide seven-tenths of 1 percent of its GNP to international development. With slow world growth, this will be hard to achieve. As we know, a heavily indebted developing world will be hard-pressed to borrow enough money to generate enough wealth internally unless direct assistance is forthcoming and spent wisely. This is a reality we cannot avoid.

Confronting Critical Global Issues

There are three commanding, sensitive, and closely interrelated issues that both rich and poor must confront if a successful new world order is to emerge. I am talking, of course, about population, environment, and health care. A fourth critical issue, the adequacy of global and local food supply, is largely dependent upon the interactions of these three variables and the constructive interdependence of nations outlined above.

Populations

As to population, as nations develop, birthrates invariably recede—another reason why promoting economic development is in our long-term interest. Nonetheless, long-standing religious and social pressures will continue to make it difficult to curb population growth to the extent necessary to relieve pressures on both human health and the global environment. It is sobering to realize that if current projections hold, the 1990s will produce the largest generation yet born—with some 1.5 billion children entering an already crowded world.

Population growth, by definition, tends to reduce standards of living except in nations that enjoy remarkable economic growth. Population growth also adds to environmental pressure—most directly, in areas where new deserts are created as forests are destroyed to provide land for cultivation. Such growth encourages exploitation of children, migrants, and others in the workplace. It pits neighboring countries against each other as they feel each other's population pressures.

It will take political courage, but leaders of both developed and developing nations must commit themselves to population planning programs as an integral part of their plans for economic development. A good place to start would be for the United States to renew its funding of the UN Fund for Population Activities.

Environment

In contrast to population, the related issue of the environment is on everyone's mind. But the question remains: Are we willing to invest the political and financial capital required to both restore and protect the health of the planet?

In the rush to development, humanity has already done irreversible damage to the planet. And both developed and developing countries are to blame.

More than half of Africa's arable land is at risk of becoming desert. One-third of Asia's and one-fifth of Latin America's land is in the same state. We learn daily of the environmental catastrophe that exists in the former Soviet Union and in much of Eastern and Central Europe. We are aware, however, that further damage can be checked and some of the prior damage reversed, if we muster the political will to act.

Various ideas for future progress are already in place. Debt-for-environment swaps permit host countries to receive debt relief in return for protecting vital environmental resources. The Global Environmental Facility created by the UN and the World Bank has helped to raise public consciousness and to offer practical alternatives. There is an emerging international consensus that environmental impact assessments should be built in to economic development plans at both national and international levels.

Issues of global warming and ozone depletion, already high on the international agenda, must not be shunned or postponed simply because they are politically difficult. To come to grips with these challenges, the nations of the Northern Hemisphere alone will need to reduce emissions of carbon dioxide from the combustion of oil, coal, and other fossil fuels by perhaps 50% in the next twenty-five years or so. And we must eliminate the use of chlorofluorocarbons—or CFCs—and halons on a far more rapid and comprehensive scale than we have so far committed ourselves to.

The scope of the problem is illustrated by the stark fact that if just four industrializing countries—India, Brazil, China, and Indo-China—were to increase their use of CFCs and halons up to the limit now permitted under the 1987 Montreal Protocol, the annual release of CFCs would increase by 40% rather than diminish.

Unfortunately, the 1992 UN Conference on Environment and

Development was a more rhetorical than substantive success, in no small part hampered by the reactionary position of the United States. Yet the conference did provide an important beginning for change, much as the Helsinki Conference on Human Rights did some years ago. The industrialized countries must take the hard choices of environmental protection if they are to have any hope of persuading the poorer nations to join in.

Providing Adequate Global Health Care

Any new world order must also include provision for adequate global health care. Dazzling accounts of organ transplantation and manipulation of the human genome fill our newspapers and periodicals. Yet, despite giant strides in medical research and development, the global delivery of adequate health care is lagging woefully behind ever-increasing demand. Complaints of failing health care systems are voiced daily around the world. In many countries we hear predictions that health care is rapidly becoming the number-one problem and that many of us, lay persons and doctors alike, are failing to meet our human responsibilities and the challenges at hand.

The facts are clear. In the United States we continue to face such long-standing problems as heart disease and cancer. In addition, newer scourges, such as AIDS and widespread international drug abuse, beset us. And new challenges, such as providing maximum functioning and independence to rapidly expanding elderly populations, test our skills and political will. On the other side of the coin, difficulties in delivering adequate medical care to expanding infant populations, especially those in our own inner cities, continue to hobble us. We have yet to demonstrate maintenance of effort in the long haul.

However, in the developing nations of the world, where health statistics document the growing disparity between the haves and have-nots, there is a gulf that divides the world of North from South as effectively as the East-West separation of the Cold War years. Throughout the tropics schistosomiasis, river blindness, pneumonia, and dysentery continue to cripple and kill. We have shown that great strides forward are possible: childhood immunizations, oral rehydration therapy for diarrhea, the conquest of smallpox – but unfortunately, we can balance tales of success with numerous failures.

Infant mortality and life expectancy rates in the developing world must be analyzed not merely as cold numbers in columns; they represent the tragic wastage of human lives, dreams, and potential in countries that can ill afford such a constant loss. AIDS is decimating whole areas of central Africa, disproportionately destroying the young, educated urban hope of that continent. In some areas over 30% of the entire population is infected with the fatal human immunodeficiency virus. There has been a resurgence of ancient scourges, with drug-resistant tuberculosis and malaria, as well as cholera, once again reaching epidemic proportions in Africa, Asia, and Latin America. Eradication and control schemes are paralyzed by lack of funds and an adequate cadre of skilled health workers.

And let no one think that these problems will be long confined to the developing nations of the world; infectious diseases simply do not recognize political borders, and the speed and frequency of air travel have broken the old quarantine barriers against contagious transmission.

We also confront the vexing issuing of skyrocketing medical costs and the fact that those who suffer most are located not only in the developing countries but also among the poor, including the working poor, in the United States. There can be no doubt that providing decent and humane medical assistance, particularly to the less-fortunate, will be a most pressing issue in any new world order. For all these reasons, we must take the necessary actions to close the existing gap. But what should we do? Recognizing the importance and complexity of these issues, let me, as a layperson, offer a few suggestions.

First, we must put increased emphasis on exploring the linkages among health care, population, and environment.

On population, I make three suggestions:

1) Strengthen biomedical research on human reproduction.

2) Strengthen psychosocial research on human reproduction.

3) Foster incorporation of family planning into health services, especially in the field of primary care.

One vehicle for the achievement of all these objectives would be to broaden and invigorate the Human Reproduction Programme of the World Health Organization.

Second, as to environment, absent careful control of the way in which growth takes place, there are often negative environmental repercussions that adversely affect human health. Examples include lead poisoning; asbestosis; inadequate sanitation; and the direct and indirect threats to health posed by poorly planned, overcrowded urban environments. There are also potential dangers to health from larger environmental problems, such as damage to the ozone layer, toxic wastes, and the incalculable long-term consequences of damage to the ecosystems of the world's great oceans.

Unfortunately, at the UN Conference on Environment and Development, there was not a clear and strong call for significantly increased health-related research backed by concrete proposals for international collaboration. It goes without saying that assuring adequate funding is also essential.

Third, as to health care systems, I believe the international community must increasingly share experience and information on the comparative advantages and disadvantages of various systems, with a view to containing health care costs without compromising access to, and the quality of, medical care.

Health care is a fundamental human need, and access to it is a fundamental human right. It must not be a privilege of the élite. Therefore, ways of providing access without generating unacceptable costs must be re-examined intensively and put into place.

In our own country excellent health care is often available to those who can pay for it. However, more than thirty million Americans have no medical insurance coverage whatsoever. This means that they do not receive care; they take their chances with charity care, or they exhaust their very meager savings.

Further, for many years health care costs in the United States have risen at a rate more than twice that of general inflation, and neither the private nor the public sector can allow this to continue. Retired people are losing their benefits, working people are making do with reduced benefits, and many small-business employers offer no health insurance coverage. The American public policy community presently is trying to find answers; but all the alternatives are crushingly expensive, and both the White House and Congress are deadlocked on what to do.

Most Western nations seem dissatisfied with their own systems, and many poor nations have no effective system at all. Each nation seems to stumble, by trial and error, through a succession of failures and shortfalls until it adopts a system that in the end is still not satisfactory. This will not do. The world community can and must demonstrate the political will necessary to develop effective systems, at acceptable costs, and with accessible services distributed equitably within societies.

Further to the point that adequate health care is both a fundamental need and a human right, I suggest that doctors could be more active in addressing issues of health promotion and disease prevention as they relate to the wider national and world communities. If we are to contribute effectively to the urgent health needs of poor nations, we cannot merely transfer our elaborate, curative medical technology. It is an inappropriate system in many other lands and distracts from the basic public health needs of most developing countries. We must learn to put greater emphasis on sanitation and nutrition, safe water supplies, and basic education and vaccination programs—projects that may not be as dramatic as disaster relief efforts but hold the only hope for long-term improvement.

Governor Dean of Vermont, himself a physician, has emphasized that doctors analytical skills and knowledge are badly needed in public life. He is not talking about the understandable need for doctors to organize to protect themselves against matters such as possible malpractice actions. Rather, he is talking about the need for doctors to take a more active role in the public processes concerned with satisfying the basic right of each individual to receive adequate health care. As we all know, good health not only affects the well-being of those who are fortunate enough to enjoy it; it also generates expanded productivity and enhanced economic growth and stability.

Finally, it should be noted that health and humanitarian assistance can be an effective tool in preventive diplomacy, not only providing immediate life-saving help, but offering a common ground that can sometimes open the difficult doors to political negotiation. There is much sustained work to be done by both medical personnel and laypersons in addressing a wide range of serious health-related problems. To do so will require a level of cooperation among different sectors of society rarely achieved.

Fostering Democracy And Human Rights

There is yet another issue that all too often is ignored. It is the erroneous belief that the internal affairs of other nations are not a proper subject for state-to-state discourse, and that internal events in other countries, such as human rights violations, are not our concern. I strongly disagree. Although our options may at times be limited in dealing with such questions, we should never stop trying to apply diplomatic, economic, and political pressures that will help the human family continue its passage toward a more open, more democratic, and freer life.

Those countries that have attempted to create economic development in a totalitarian framework have found it does not work. The human spirit, liberated, is capable of productivity and achievement undreamed of under the deadening hand of conformist control. We have seen that economic and social policy steps contribute to development—the establishment of constitutional government, the rule of law, accountability of government officials, openness, and respect for human rights.

Moreover, I believe that, just as the United Nations should establish early-warning mechanisms to foresee and, if possible, forestall military conflict between nations, the UN must continue to expand and strengthen its machinery for monitoring and bringing pressure to bear on violations of political and human rights.

As I mentioned above, the tragic ethnic conflicts that devastated Yugoslavia, parts of the former Soviet Union, and are still rife among other countries—Somalia and the Congo—are, at core, egregious violations of political human rights.

The tide of history is not running in the wrong direction. Although some events are currently beyond our control, the tide still flows toward openness and freedom of the individual—concepts that lie at the heart of many religious and ethical traditions around the world.

Strengthening the Key International Institutions

In the 1940s the international community held historic summits in San Francisco and Bretton Woods that helped establish a basis for a more enlightened world order. The Stockholm Initiative, to which I referred earlier, proposes that a comparable world summit on global governance be called to address the unprecedented challenges and opportunities that confront us today.

Such a global summit, which would have to be very carefully prepared through a process of consultation and negotiation among the participants, would, I suspect, lead not only the United States but most nations to the realization that it is incumbent on us to modernise institutions of cooperation – and to create new or modified instructions where needed. Much has been done to modernize, streamline, and strengthen the United Nations to meet the tasks that face it. There must be ongoing efforts to broaden the UN's mandate at the Security Council level, strengthen the authority of the Secretary-General, and continue to improve and stabilize the UN financial system.

I have suggested several structural changes that could be steps on the road to greater international peace and security; to shared and sustainable economic development; to curbing uncontrolled population growth and environmental degradation: to providing adequate global health care: to fostering democracy and human rights; and to creating a world order in which both law and justice become the norm, rather than the exception.

As we rush toward our date with the millennium, we have, I believe, an unparalleled chance to define that future.

Let us seize the moment.

The Royal College of Surgeons in Ireland

The Royal College of Surgeons in Ireland (RCSI), founded in 1784 to certify surgical training, established a medical school in the mid 19th century. By the time Ireland became an independent country in 1922, a tradition had been established of accepting students from many countries throughout the world. In the mid 20th century, the leadership of RCSI, under Dr. Harry O'Flanagan, adopted an entry mechanism whereby one third of the students were from developed countries, one third were from developing countries, and one third from Ireland.

Today, RCSI is an independent, not-for-profit, health sciences institution with a unique international perspective.

Its undergraduate medical school is the largest in Ireland. As demand for places increased substantially in the late 20th century, the capacity within Dublin was exhausted. At that stage, RCSI established two medical campuses in Malaysia, and one in Bahrain. Additional non-medical school campuses have also been established in Dubai and Abu Dhabi.

The College continually invests in educational standards, innovations and facilities in order to provide internationally recognised and respected medical and health sciences qualifications. RCSI is by Government Statute an independent, degree–awarding body in Ireland. It is also a recognised College of the National University of Ireland.

The mission of RCSI is "To educate, nurture and discover for the benefit of human health".

The Center for International Humanitarian Cooperation and the Institute of International Humanitarian Affairs

The Center for International Humanitarian Cooperation (CIHC) is a U.S. registered public charity that was founded in 1992 to promote healing and peace in countries shattered by natural disasters, armed conflicts, and ethnic violence. The Center employs its resources and unique personal contacts to stimulate interest in humanitarian issues and to promote innovative educational programs and training models.

Our extensive list of publications and regular symposia address both the basic issues and the emerging challenges of humanitarian assistance. Since 2001 the CIHC has supported training in humanitarian issues through the Institute of International Humanitarian Affairs at Fordham University (IIHA); it has now educated over 2300 humanitarian aid professionals from 133 nations, and continues to offer programs in Europe, Asia, Africa, Latin America and North America. The CIHC has formal partnerships with the Royal College of Surgeons in Ireland, University College Dublin, the NOHA network of European universities, United Nations World Food Programme (WFP), International Organization of Migration (IOM), International Medical Corps (IMC), Action Contre La Faim (ACF), Jesuit Refugee Service (JRS), the British Ministry of Defense, and other UN, NGO and governmental organizations. For more information, please refer to our website www.cihc.org

International Humanitarian Affairs (IHA) Book Series

The IHA series, written or edited by Kevin M. Cahill, M.D., is devoted to improving the effectiveness of humanitarian relief programs. With contributions by leading professionals, the books are practical guides to responding to the many different effects of civil strife, natural disasters, epidemics, and other crises. All books are available online at www.fordhampress.com.

Books marked with an asterisk are available in French translation from Robert Laffont of Paris.

Preventive Diplomacy: Stopping Wars Before They Start, 2000*

Basics of International Humanitarian Missions, 2003*

Emergency Relief Operations, 2003*

Traditions, Values, and Humanitarian Action, 2003*

Human Security for All: A Tribute to Sergio Vieira de Mello, 2004 *Technology for Humanitarian Action,* 2004

To Bear Witness: A Journey of Healing and Solidarity, 2005*

Tropical Medicine: A Clinical Text, 7th edition, 2006

The Pulse of Humanitarian Assistance, 2007

Even in Chaos: Education in Times of Emergency, 2010

Sudan at the Brink: F. D. Deng, 2010, with Foreword by Kevin M. Cahill, M.D.*

Tropical Medicine: A Clinical Text, 8th edition (Jubilee Edition), 2011*

More with Less: Disasters in an Era of Diminishing Resources, 2012

History and Hope: The International Humanitarian Reader, 2013

To Bear Witness: A Journey of Healing and Solidarity, 2nd edition, 2013